DUTY
of
CARE

DUTY

of

CARE

Dr DOMINIC PIMENTA

+ HEROES

W

WELBECK

Published by Welbeck Non-Fiction Limited,
part of Welbeck Publishing Group.
20 Mortimer Street,
London W1T 3JW

First published by Welbeck in 2020

Note: in order to preserve the absolute confidentiality of the patients in
this book, certain details, names and places have been changed or merged
where necessary.

A CIP catalogue record for this book is available from the British Library

ISBN Paperback – 9781787395596

Typeset by seagulls.net
Printed and bound in the UK.

10 9 8 7 6 5 4 3 2

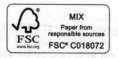

www.welbeckpublishing.com

For Dilsan, Ayla and Zach

CONTENTS

CHAPTER 1   Calm waters   1

CHAPTER 2   Exposure   21

CHAPTER 3   Incubation   51

CHAPTER 4   Symptoms   65

CHAPTER 5   Escalation   113

CHAPTER 6   Complications   165

CHAPTER 7   Critical   207

CHAPTER 8   Recovery   303

EPILOGUE   Immunity   317

ADDENDUM   335

ACKNOWLEDGEMENTS   341

ABOUT THE AUTHOR   343

CHAPTER 1

Calm waters

I have had the same recurring dream since early childhood.

I am standing on a beach, curling my toes into soft, warm sand like fine brown sugar. The sky is an endless, untouched, pristine blue. Families and couples dot the shore. Sometimes my own family is there with me – sometimes my parents, sometimes my wife and kids – and sometimes no one at all.

On the horizon, the sea and sky merge in a blurry haze. As I'm staring out across the water, something moves. I strain to see the distant event, my eyes ache and my chest knots, as the horizon lifts and swells. Bigger and bigger, a black wall of water rises and rises. Sometimes I shout and no one moves, sometimes we stampede away from the shore, sometimes I can do nothing at all. The wave gets closer and closer until it plunges the beach into darkness and fills the world. Sometimes it hits. Sometimes, just as it's about to, I wake.

This time, I wake from the dream with my heart racing well over 150 beats per minute. As a heart doctor, a cardiology registrar, I've started to wonder if this is some sort of nocturnal arrhythmia, pounding in my chest. I try the manoeuvres I ask of my patients – forcing my breath out with mouth closed and nose pinched, splashing my face with water – and even the ones I do myself, like massaging my carotid artery as it pulsates at the angle of the jaw, trying to trick the knot of autonomic nerve tissue there into resetting my heartbeat – but nothing settles it, except time.

My wife, Dilsan, mutters something and rolls over. It's 5 a.m. and my alarm is about to go off anyway. Our two kids, Ayla and Zach, could go off at any time from now until 7 as well. I get out of bed, shower, get changed. Despite my shuffling about and our creaky floors, no one is up yet. At 6.30 a.m., I'm out the door. It's the middle of January and it's still pitch-black. A brisk walk on icy concrete, pit stop at Costa, and I'm plonked on the tube, winding my way through the bowels of London to my job at a specialist heart hospital.

Trying to avoid social media, I use the hour-plus commute to learn some coding or to write, putting some words together for one of the newspapers I occasionally contribute to or some-times just jotting down some nonsense. I work on my Notes app on my phone, penning whatever the flavour of the day happens to be: a novella about a Frankenstein-like child that grows into an insatiable, power-hungry tyrant; a children's book for my daughter about a detective hunting lost triangles; or a memoir I'd mothballed after probably too few rejections. Meanwhile, the train skips and whispers through the stations.

I jump up the stairs of the hospital, usually still attached to my phone, picking up another coffee if I have a free voucher, and then through the doors to cardiology, a large unit on the top floor. I'm there at 8, or earlier, on days I'm on call. We have multiple subspecialty departments of cardiology, each a centre of excellence in its own right, and as a middle-grade doctor, half-way through specialist training, I rotate through all three. My last rotation, specialty cardiology, is where everything that doesn't involve inserting stents in heart arteries (specialized tubes designed to keep the arteries open) or dangerous heart rhythms ends up.

The handover from the previous shift takes place in a tiny room for the nurses, plus me and one doctor more junior than me, a Senior House Officer (SHO). The night nurse in charge will rattle through the list of patients – their histories and plans, any problems or updates, and who might fall or have an infection. They occasionally intersperse the handover with a joke or a jibe, usually at the expense of another hospital "tribe" – for example, referencing "difficult" radiologists, the "slow" porters or the "hard-headed" surgeons and cardiologists. Most nurses will spend their working lives on a single ward, and many of them have worked together for over a decade. They are a family of sorts. In those handovers, as junior doctors, we are ever the interlopers, and just as we begin to know names and faces, we often move on.

The handover breaks up and we start the round. The consultant (the senior doctor, who has worked their way up through their chosen specialty) for that particular week will join us most days, sometimes to see every patient and sometimes for a quicker review of the new patients. We make our way round at what an old boss would call a "physicianly" pace. "You can do medicine good, or fast," she would often say, "but you can't do both." Our professional personas are patchwork cloaks of the seniors we have learnt from and the mistakes we have made, and this one got sewn into mine. Another boss, another patch on the cloak, would always go through every single aspect of each patient every day: history, blood tests, ECG, chest X-ray, vital signs, patient symptoms, examination, plan and review. These are the examples I try to live up to, but it's a lot harder than it looks.

The patients on this ward are a hodgepodge from all over: adults with congenital heart diseases that were corrected as a baby or child with new problems arising from their original surgery; hearts dangerously infected with bacteria lodged on valves, sometimes waiting for or recovering from open-heart surgery; and patients with degenerative heart valves, failing heart muscles, genetic heart diseases or heart cancers. The youngest is sometimes as young as 17 and the oldest patient I ever looked after was 102. Every patient needs as much attention paid to their heart as to every other part of them. Their kidneys can get damaged by too little or too much fluid, and by infections, medicines or clots; their lungs can fill with fluid inside and around them; their brains can get confused or infected; and their bowels can slow down or develop clots. The complexity makes each day a marathon, but also makes every day new. I see everyone from porters to professors, coming from every part of London and beyond. They're each different but they're all humans, with unique stories to tell.

On those days, I tend to eat lunch juggling external calls about unwell patients in other hospitals and moving between wards to see internal referrals. The hours race by and 5 p.m. comes and often goes. Since I've had kids, I've tried to be much stricter about the time, handing over when my shift ends and going home. My time isn't just mine anymore – it belongs to my wife, my daughter and my son as much as anyone. I often get it wrong, though, nonetheless. Reeling off the evening jobs and the list of sick patients to the overnight doctor, I shoot out the door and back onto the tube. If I'm quick at the change-overs and barrel down the escalators I can sometimes make it for bedtime. I often don't. It's dark again by the time I'm home. Dilsan has usually had a worse day than me – two kids, middle of winter, stuck inside most of the day. We get 14 years of training to be a doctor, and about 14 minutes to be a parent. We are both doctors, we try our best, it's hard. Dinner. TV. Settle one or both kids. Bed.

•   •   •

If you asked a handful of my colleagues the question, "When did you decide to become a doctor?" I think you'd get back a handful of answers. Mine would be the dullest: I honestly can't remember ever wanting to do anything else. No one in my immediate family is medical but my mum's brother was a nurse, and we have a few doctors in the extended family on my dad's side. My dad is originally from Bombay via Nairobi, while my mum's family is Irish-English and descended from generations of British Army colonials in India. Dad left India when he was only three, in the middle of World War Two, but my maternal grandmother, Patricia, was born in Bangalore in 1935 to a British Army soldier from Ireland. All our stories of growing up in India came from her: panthers prowling on the veranda, Gurkhas digging the family out of heavy snowfalls in the Kashmiri mountains and chapatis being snatched from her hand by wild eagles – which she had the scar to prove. With feet planted in several cultures, I never really felt like I truly belonged to one. Through school and then college, there was always a sense of "otherness". I remember a handful of racist incidents growing up – older boys harassing me and my brother in the park, and getting shouted at in my first job in the dairy aisle at Tesco for running out of milk by a red-faced, green-tweed-clad denizen of some country pile, who opened with "You Muslims are all the same!" (I'm not Muslim, but that is beside the point).

When I finally reached medical school, I found a sense of belonging. Medicine, with its unique vernacular, rites of passage, arcane knowledge and long-held traditions, is a tribe of its own. I loved medical school, from the dissection room to the lecture theatre to the teaching ward rounds, and finally felt at home.

Most importantly, I met my wife in our very first year. At the time I was supposed to be raising money for the medical school charity, running a street collection in fancy dress. The first time I ever saw Dilsan I was wearing a suit of golden armour, which was actually badly spray-painted cardboard boxes, so terribly put together that bits would occasionally fly off and a friend would have to tape them back on again. The early January weather was arctic, and underneath this flimsy cardboard covering I was just wearing a t-shirt and shorts. If I'd known then that I was about to meet the woman I'd spend the rest of my life with, I would probably have taken more care with my outfit. Up until that point, I didn't believe in love at first sight, or even love per se. But from the moment I saw her, wearing a much more sensible outfit, plus fairy wings and a crown, I instantly believed in both. We've been together ever since. An artist and now a general surgical registrar and academic, Dilsan is my better half, in every sense of the word.

To make sure we didn't get separated in our first jobs as doctors, we applied together, and ended up on the same exact rotations: Slough, and then Oxford. My first ever day as a doctor, I did a ward round of about 10 very stable vascular surgery patients completely alone, called my seniors about every minor blood result and went home exhausted with anxiety despite, in retrospect, nothing having happened whatsoever. The step from student to doctor is a chasm. After spending years as the shadow to actual doctors, you one day find yourself as the real deal. The safety net feels like it's been swept away, and you are holding the weight of responsibility in your hands alone, teetering on the brink of disaster. Of course, we aren't usually alone, with extended teams above and around us and our junior colleagues going through the same baptism of fire. There isn't a closer feeling of camaraderie in medicine than in those first few months, when bonds of friendship are made that persist years after. The other first-year doctors we worked with were at our wedding; we've held their newborn children and they've held ours. But over time, rotations and hospitals come and go, and it becomes harder and harder to make and maintain those connections. As you get more senior, you work consistently with fewer and fewer people, and your teams dwindle to sometimes just you. It isn't until you put down roots as a consultant that you can start to make those long-term working relationships again, but the road there is long and often lonely.

I've been a doctor for eight years now. I struggled in those early days to find a specialty that fitted; I always wanted to do hospital medicine but bounced between infectious disease, intensive care and then finally cardiology. In those first rotations as an F1 (standing for Foundation Year 1, the first year after you graduate from med school and are placed in a hospital), I'd spent four months working in microbiology. I had an office in the pathology lab, literally among the microscopes and agar plates, where I'd sit and process reports of bacteria, viruses and other bugs and then wander round the wards with the consultant, matching reports to people. We saw some strange things, in a hospital very close to an international airport. Infections in general account for one in four of every emergency admission to hospital, and my favourite part of the day would be the rounds in intensive care. Rare infections of the brain, listeriosis, devastating infections of the skin and soft tissue, necrotizing fasciitis and even a case of very rare infection and reaction from abroad in a patient with leptospirosis. Our days were filled by diagnostic conundrums. I'd spend weeks phoning special testing units for results on tropical or super-rare diseases and carrying still-warm tissue specimens around the hospital in my pocket to courier directly to the lab. It was the weirdest and best job I did in those early years.

Much later on in my medical rotations I worked in a proper tropical diseases hospital, where my bosses included Professor Chris Whitty, no less. One of the best jobs I've ever worked was manning the tropical disease walk-in clinic, a clinic exclusively for travellers returning from abroad. We saw lots of dengue fever, some infected hearts (endocarditis) and lots of people who believed they had worm infections – and one, at least, who definitely did, as became clear when he coughed up an 8-cm ascaris worm into his hand in the waiting room. For a while, this was where I wanted to stay.

I remembered those days fondly in 2019 when I heard that Professor Whitty had become Chief Medical Officer for the UK government. I doubt he'll remember me, but his rounds were unforgettable. We used to present our cases from the tropical disease clinic on a Friday morning. Coffee plus pastry plus a menagerie of microscopic critters from all over the world equals happiness. We'd present the cases in the same format:

"I saw a 50-year-old man from Malawi."

"STOP!" he'd pronounce, in that authoritative but jovial voice. "Diseases from Malawi. Go!" And we'd buzz round the table describing as many infectious diseases from Malawi as possible.

At the time, Professor Whitty was sitting on the COBRA meetings about the Ebola crisis, and we'd joke that he'd probably cut off the then Prime Minister David Cameron with a "STOP!", and then quiz the Cabinet in the same way. He is a brilliant and decent man and an incredible teacher. He also has a law degree, just for fun. When he was appointed Chief Medical Officer, I couldn't think of a better person for the job, and I still think that.

Meanwhile, my career plans drifted from infectious diseases when, in my fourth year as a doctor, I chose to work in intensive care. Where we worked, the patient load was split mostly between routine surgical patients recovering from operations, and very unwell blood cancer patients, often young adults and even teenagers. By a quirk of the rota I seemed to find myself constantly carrying out rounds on these desperately sick young men and women. I remember that time as perpetual night: it was winter rotation and I would leave home before the sun was up and get back home long after it had set. At the shift handovers we would carefully go through the numbers, the mechanical metrics of a human being on life support: ventilator settings, the relative amounts of gases in the blood (oxygen and CO_2, measured sometimes hourly in intensive care), the blood pressure and drugs needed to keep them there, the amount of urine produced per hour and the blood test results. Abnormal was the norm for those patients, with blood counts sometimes in the single figures – they had no cells to clot, so there was a risk of developing torrential bleeds, and with no cells to fight infection, there was always the chance of contracting overwhelming infections. These patients, like most intensive care patients, are complex and fragile, and need meticulous daily attention to keep inching ever in the right direction. Too often, though, they would go in the wrong direction.

Despite the sometimes crushing environment, I really enjoyed intensive care. The stakes were incredibly high, the medicine as much an art as a science, and everything felt vital and important. What I also discovered about myself was that I really enjoyed doing things: like putting in lines in arteries or veins and helping to put tubes in lungs and chests. These were small triumphs, but gave a sense of accomplishment, of control, when so much else was failure and we were powerless to prevent it. ICU held a practical and beautiful complexity for me; the highs of snatching a patient from the jaws of death were stratospheric, but the lows were subterranean. I worried that the emotional and physical strain of the work was making me a terrible husband – grumpy, tired and prone to outbursts. I remember on the way to one night shift – the third consecutive shift in a group of four, with little sleep in between – my walk to the tube seemed particularly leaden. We'd lost one patient the night before, a 17-year-old girl, and looked likely to lose another in the next 48 hours. Earphones in, hunched in the tube, something twitched and I found myself in tears for the entire journey. I couldn't really explain why but felt all the better for it when I got to handover. I'm not very good at emotions – I find it hard to connect the inner and outer spheres. Some of the best doctors I ever met were lifelong ICU doctors. How my colleagues stayed sane in those careers, I won't ever know. I was and remain in awe of them.

What eventually captured my heart, so to speak, was cardiology, the medicine of the heart. Of all the human organs, the heart is hands-down the best. As a cardiologist you might think I'm quite biased, but, respectfully, history is firmly on my side. In Ancient Greece, Aristotle thought the heart was the "seat and soul" of human consciousness, famously dismissing the brain as merely for "cooling of the blood". (That's the skin, by the way.) Galen, a fellow Ancient Greek physician whose ideas would inform European medicine for centuries, believed the heart was the physical site of a "tripartite soul", with the brain and spleen of equal importance.

It's not clear why the heart was so recognized as the organ of essential importance that its very name became synonymous with the idea of something central and essential. It was noted throughout ancient history that the quickest way to kill a human being was to injure their heart. As with most of human discovery, perhaps the earliest advance in our understanding that the heart was the life-giving centre came from war and violence.

The heart has historically been a bedrock of culture and religion since time immemorial, reflected in the ubiquity of the heart in our day-to-day parlance. You can have a change of heart, have your "heartstrings" pulled or your heart "set aflutter". Hearts can be cold, closed, empty or black. They can be worn on our sleeves and given away. They can even be "broken", which is more than just a figurative term. A fairly recent discovery, "broken heart syndrome" (formally called Takotsubo cardiomyopathy, named after the shape of an octopus trap used by Japanese fishermen) is rare and generally occurs after a major life event or massive upset. The first time I ever saw this was in a patient of mine who fell and broke her hip while planning her husband's funeral. The results from blood tests (which look specifically for a protein that is released if the heart muscle is damaged) were so unusual that the lab phoned me directly. Suspecting a heart attack, an ultrasound of her heart was scheduled for the next morning. As I looked over the technician's shoulder, she pointed out the problem: while the normal heart should be a muscular, rounded oblong, tapering gently to a point at the apex, each segment contracting and relaxing in perfect synchrony, the heart before me looked very different, ballooned and thinned at the apex into a bubble of flesh that barely moved at all. It was extraordinary: I was staring at the physical manifestation of a broken heart. Our hearts are so inextricably linked to our minds that it made me wonder if Galen didn't have it right all along: inside our hearts rests a little bit of our souls as well.

For such a cultural touchstone, the heart was an organ we really didn't know very much about for a very long time. If all of human history from 6000 BC to 2020 AD was a single day, it's only in the last 20 minutes or so we've really had any fathomable clue of the function and mechanics of what is our most vital organ (although I may again be guilty of bias here). In fact, keeping to our analogy here, the advances have been so rapid and so recent that the whole field has been transformed in a matter of seconds.

It's rare in medicine to be truly hands-on, to "fix" someone. Cardiology is different – we do these things all the time. We put wires and stents in heart arteries, heart valves and heart chambers, inserting pacemakers and electrodes to make the heart speed up when it's too slow or delivering energy to burn away areas of tissue that are causing the heart to beat too quickly. We handle heart transplants and even give patients artificial hearts. Some surgeries are just remarkable, like grafting a transplanted heart onto a failing one instead of swapping it, leaving the patient with two physical hearts and two separate heart beats, a condition called "piggyback" heart.

I finished core medical training and became a cardiology specialist registrar in 2016, shortly before our first child, Ayla, was born. I had a dream of a year off, having weekends back and reconnecting with friends and family. This easy life seemed all set, until Dilsan pointed out that there was a baby due imminently and bills to pay. Scrambling for a job, I applied for a non-training registrar post in cardiology at a local district general hospital. I loved it straight away – it was everything I had wanted to escape as a junior: the endless paperwork, gruelling tick-box exercises and hoop-jumping around the department for "sign-offs" disappeared. I didn't have a login for the computer for three months and it was wonderful. Suddenly it was pure medicine again: see a patient, listen to their story, examine them, make a diagnosis and treat them. It was also exhilaratingly terrifying.

I remember once asking a brand-new consultant on their first day what it felt like, and he told me, "like driving a very very fast car: it's fun, but also scary as hell". Being a brand-new registrar was exactly like that. It's easy to fall into a cul-de-sac, circling the monotony of endless ward rounds as a junior. But this felt like the open road, and I was excited but fearful as well. I wrote down notes about every single patient I saw or discussed for four weeks, and would ask my incredibly understanding consultants, in what must have been excruciating detail, if they were happy with every decision.

The other great thing about that very first job was that I didn't do anything else; I didn't work weekends or nights, and I didn't go to other training areas or study days or rotate anywhere. Every single day for nearly a year, I just saw cardiology patients – we would see around 20 ward patients and then 15–20 ward referrals every day. I was there for such a long time that I developed something we hardly ever get in hospital medicine training: patient continuity. I can remember a handful of patients I saw many times, one of whom, during our fourth and fifth encounter, joked that I was his "personal cardiologist", while another more waspish patient would greet me on our repeat encounters with a forceful "you again?!" It's actually very rare in training to ever get to see the long- or even mid-term outcomes of your actions, like the patient with chest pain that you just felt wasn't quite right and decided to admit, to find three days later that their main coronary artery was hanging on by a thread, a whisper away from a possibly fatal heart attack. This job was a constant carousel of my decisions revisited; the wins were incredibly rewarding and the failures were the best training I've ever had. I was fortunate to have great bosses, and enough time to learn.

At the end of that year I got into the cardiology training programme and moved to a large general hospital with an advanced heart service. I thought I'd be well prepared, but this was another level, and as a trainee there was far more to do procedurally, which came with its own terrain of joys and challenges. I thought I knew what busy was, but the on-call shifts were some of the most intense I've ever worked. A single registrar would cover emergency patients arriving by both the front door (A&E) and the back door (the direct heart attack service), the cardiology wards at night and all the referrals across 10 floors of busy specialist care, on top of receiving referrals from a whole other district general hospital without specialist heart services. Those shifts were sometimes brutal, a physical and mental battle, without any of the support networks I'd known before. The first year of proper cardiology training was like a forge – I felt white-hot and beaten into shape, with a few dents to show for it. I took away a phenomenal amount, and, after two years, in 2018, I finally landed at the large tertiary heart centre where I work today.

Around the time Dilsan became pregnant again, in autumn 2018, we were living in Tottenham in north-east London. We were only five doors down from her sister, Neslisan, and her husband Ehsan, who we are very close with. Nes is a teacher and Ehsan works in IT for several large schools, and we are perpetually jealous of their long holidays. Their children are only a little older than ours, and we would spend most of our weekends and days off together. On the incredibly rare moments that we could get all the kids asleep in one house, we would try to spend an evening as well: a movie, perhaps a board game, but not Monopoly, which is now banned following an incident that we no longer speak of. Dilsan and I, both being doctors, would occasionally get calls when their oldest was a baby and would get ill, and we'd sprint up the street in pyjamas to try and reassure the new parents. Ironically, when we had Ayla, we would call them for the exact same reasons. The cousins all growing up together is the best life I could want for them.

Fairly broke after one child and a year of full-time extortionate nursery fees, we tried to look for a place to move to have a second. Lots of back and forth followed, but the tipping point came not by a house we fell in love with, but rather by the appearance of a dead body in our street after someone experienced an overdose at a newly opened crack den just one street over. We had to step round the police cordon to get to our front door.

"What's that?" asked Ayla.

"It's the reason we're moving house," came my clipped reply.

We put in an offer we couldn't afford the very next day and moved further north.

To pay the bills during Dilsan's maternity I'd been working two jobs. Day-to-day, I was a trainee heart doctor, about three years at a push from reaching consultancy, at the specialist heart hospital. My second job was more of the same at other hospitals in London, ad hoc general medicine agency shifts on weekends and on days off.

Despite my love of cardiology, on top of the usual satellite clinics (owned by the hospital but operated on another site), heart CT or MRI scanning sessions and the regular on-calls, the extra hours doing agency shifts were starting to take a toll. Trying to balance home life, work life and all the paperwork between was becoming overwhelming. Deflated and in need of a break from clinical medicine, I started making plans to take a temporary hiatus from cardiology into what has become a nearly obligatory part of training: to go and do a PhD or MD. It's perfectly possible to traverse the entirety of cardiology training without doing a research degree, but the vast majority of trainees will, which makes consultant posts nearly impossible to obtain without one, at least in London.

The subject that came to mind was the use of artificial intelligence in cardiology. As a somewhat headstrong and possibly slightly obnoxious teenager, when I applied to study medicine at four medical schools – the maximum number you can apply to – I also applied to do a course in AI. Of course, not bothering to write a new application for this course, I didn't get accepted on it. And then, as the years went by, AI went from a novelty on a UCAS application form to a ubiquitous and vital part of modern human life, and everywhere I looked in cardiology some new AI algorithm or technique was popping up.

• • •

As January 2020 began, it coincided with a dark time in my life, both figuratively and literally. Zach (just six months old) wasn't sleeping, our maternity pay was about to run out entirely, and everyone was tetchy and tired and stretched. I'd just burnt myself out on social media over the election period. Thankfully, two things happened. Firstly, my brother (Paul) booked a surprise holiday to London from the USA over Christmas. We hadn't seen each other for nearly three years, and I'd only ever met his oldest child. I brined a turkey, took two weeks off, ate my own weight in chocolate, and dashed around half of London's sights with my kids and nieces. My younger sister, Beck, lived with us over the holiday and planned an elaborate surprise for my parents, who had no idea my brother was going to turn up to Christmas dinner from 10,000 miles away. Speaking with my cardiology hat on, I was quite against the idea of initiating a huge shock, given that my dad, Leander, is an Indian man (and thus prone to coronary heart disease) and over 80 years old (although he is pretty fit and, incredibly, still working, despite my protestations). My mum, Debbie, 20 years his junior, would be a blubbering mess but would be fine. After a few weeks of intense discussion, I lost the argument and we kept them both in the dark. Thankfully, the day before, somehow Dad managed to find out anyway, but it was still a magical moment to be all together, with all my mum's grandchildren, for the first time ever.

The second thing that happened was that I threw my phone away. I put it in a box by the front door, and there it stayed. Social media fools your brain with all the right social cues and impulses, but it doesn't feed your soul like those actual interactions should; it's like junk food for your mind. I went on a digital detox. I felt nearly instantly better. I started to be more positive, and took stock of what was really important in my life.

So with my newly self-enforced social media ban, I diverted the time to an online qualification studying machine learning and started exploring the uncertain winds of academia to go and see what I could make of AI and hearts. I also loved spending time learning how to code. It was like a head-bangingly hard puzzle that suddenly became simple once you knew the trick. The learning curve was steep but satisfying, and I could load up the exercises on my laptop and park myself in the corner of a tube carriage while I completed them. Consumed again, this time by finishing the course, applying for research jobs and trying to barter for time away to actually do a PhD, the outside world was passing me by. On top of all that, we had a whole catalogue of issues with the new house – faulty electrics, gas supply and drain, and damp – and I had a bank account to keep out of the red and a family to support. At the time, the biggest disaster of the day was invariably poo-related. I started running again and trying to eat better. Life was busy, but good.

CHAPTER 2

Exposure

I'm not sure where my nightmare of the approaching tsunami comes from, but I know I would have it nearly daily when we went on holiday. Whenever we went to the beach my dad would stand thigh-high in the sea and throw us, shrieking with laughter, over the titanic waves we would sometimes get. In my memory these waves were 10 ft tall or more, walls of water that we would so narrowly escape. Later, my brother and I would jump headfirst into these seemingly colossal plumes, letting the force propel us toward the shore. We loved it.

During the last year of medical school, it's traditional to go and study for at least part of the year in another country. Some students will go and do a higher module in an area of special interest; others will go and work in a different healthcare setting to understand how medicine is practised around the world. Dilsan and I took our medical school elective abroad in Samoa. It was an eye-opening experience, a clash of Western and traditional Pacific cultures, with the two very different sets of health problems that each of those brought. I saw things I doubt I'll see ever again in my lifetime: gout so terrible a man's hands were unrecognizable, with calcified deposits known as tophi that just looked like a bunch of rocks attached to his wrists; a young woman dying of a mysterious illness we thought might be "wet beriberi", a fatal lack of the vitamin thiamine, caused by pregnancy-related vomiting for months without treatment. Stray dogs slept in the baking midday sun outside the ICU, and we would end most days sitting on the beach in our scrubs, watching the most beautiful sunsets. It was a surreal and deeply wonderful experience.

One night we stayed on the sister island of Savai'i. At least that was the plan. In a hut on the beach I lay down wide awake, listening maniacally to the whisper of the waves coming in and out, in and out, but then out once more? Was that the first trough of a tsunami? In the pitch-black night, the sky ablaze with stars, I was on the beach again, trying to stare out at the horizon. After the third time I think Dilsan suggested we left. We were on the 5 a.m. boat back to the mainland. I'd like to tell you that this was a one-off, but a few years later I was doing it again, on a holiday in Tenerife of all places, checking the volcanic activity of nearby Gran Canaria, waiting for the wave.

And then one Christmas, Dilsan and I were curled up on the couch. I'd just come down from settling one of the kids, and a movie was just starting on the TV. I'd missed the titles, but it was set in Thailand and Ewan McGregor was ushering two kids around a coastal hotel resort. Quite soon afterward, I was watching my nightmare unfold in HD widescreen – a crashing tidal wave wiped out the hotel complex, as the family and thousands of others were caught helplessly in its wake. I realized that it was the film *The Impossible*, and I was livid at first, because I'd heard about it and had been trying to avoid watching it for years, but Dilsan insisted we continue through to the end. It helped, briefly. I'm not a particularly anxious or irrational person, in fact usually quite the opposite, but I have never been able to shake that feeling, that cold knot, warning of impending doom, once I get it.

* * *

My brother Paul lived in China for years, in Xining and then Shanghai, an eight-hour drive from Wuhan. He moved there when we were in our early twenties, and then stayed out there before moving to Los Angeles a few years ago. It still seems such a wild concept that he could move to a city larger than London that I'd never heard of, but, to the citizens of Xining, Paul was an equally wild concept, a foreigner living in a city with nearly no tourists whatsoever. I'd never heard of Wuhan either, before the outbreak started.

One cold evening, Dilsan looked up from her phone.

"Did you hear about this thing in China? It's killed 10 people, it says here."

I snorted into my tea. "Where's that? Facebook? Fake NEWS."

"This is CNN."

"Oh."

The details were vague, a "mystery virus" in the city of Wuhan, China. It sounded like some sort of food infection reported as a local outbreak around a meat market. I knew that Ebola and other serious viruses could be transmitted through bodily fluids from animals. I read the article Dilsan handed to me and passed back her phone.

"Huh. Interesting. Wonder what that was."

I went back to messing up some very simple code and swearing loudly.

Those first reports of outbreaks of coronavirus I remember reading with academic dispassion. In my career I'd seen a few of these global viral epidemics, looked after plenty of cases of swine flu and bird flu, and lots of dengue fever. Just the year prior we had had a particularly nasty strain of influenza in the UK that seemed to like heart muscles, and we saw many heart attacks and even Takotsubos in the weeks after an infection. Even more recently, just a few months before, we had had a strange run of (probably) viral heart infections. There were four or five patients with myocarditis, essentially inflamed heart muscles, desperately young and desperately sick, with hearts prone to suddenly pause or to jump into life-threatening rhythms. They all arrived within three days of each other, and two within 45 minutes, direct to my ward. Both were barely out of their teenage years, jumping in and out of heart-stopping rhythms, and nearly every blood result came back wildly abnormal, a screen of row after row flashing in red. All of them ended up in intensive care. Huddled in our team discussing the cases with the ICU doctors, it felt like a mini-epidemic, and we discussed declaring it to Public Health England if a sixth patient appeared. That sixth patient never arrived and, fortunately, all of the five survived, but even that short run gave me a now all-too-familiar sinking feeling, as if we were being overrun.

Five years ago, I saw the only other serious possible coronavirus patient I'd ever seen. She was a young lady, just off the plane from Qatar, who was feverish and barely able to breathe.

She had suspected MERS (Middle East Respiratory Syndrome), a cousin of the coronavirus we're now facing. A few years before that we'd had SARS (Severe Acute Respiratory Syndrome, also a type of coronavirus) scares when we were travelling in Bali. But these incidents simply became touchstones of interest, isolated cases and potential diagnoses to learn from. I'm not sure I ever would have recalled MERS or SARS as coronaviruses. At that time, Corona was still simply my favourite beer.

That wasn't the end to it, and further reports of "a new viral illness" kept coming. As the new disease came from a country famous for secrecy, it wasn't clear at first what the shape of the illness was, and I, like many others, didn't pay it much attention. Out of interest more than anything else, I'd occasionally dip into Google News and then the scientific research. But years of swine flu, avian flu, SARS, MERS and regular influenza made me think that this was nothing unusual. Another season, another virus, this time the Wuhan coronavirus, and in the unlikely event that it would ever come here, we would cope with the handful of cases from abroad that we might see. In the meantime, there were babies crying and bills to pay and endless paperwork to fill in.

In the midst of all this, I was trying to write. A throwaway comment from my sister Beck one day – "Whatever happened to your book? It was okay you know" – made me decide to self-publish my previously mothballed manuscript and let it loose on Amazon. Then I started writing other pieces for various newspapers. I was also trying to finish my machine-learning qualifications and put together grant proposals about the use of AI in various clinical situations. I could foresee the huge benefit of AI in my field to take over all the mundane and simple tasks where we are prone to occasionally make mistakes, through human factors of distraction and bias, rather than lack of cognitive ability. Meanwhile, my day-to-day was occupied by both trying to build algorithms to interpret images of heart stents, and processing the risk of different types of people experiencing heart attack and heart failure.

And then, as soon as I started sniffing around the research, something awoke in me. I'd spent years wondering about various clinical questions without the time or resources to pursue them. On my commute, I was writing all sorts of wild ideas, like analyzing the fingerprint of the thousands of bacteria in human faeces with AI to identify patterns linked to obesity and to work out who should eat what and how much to avoid heart disease and stroke. With the prospect of a paid research job and time on the horizon, my brain was alight with possible futures. It's that feeling you get as a kid when you are allowed to run free and explore a new space.

As the coronavirus blew through Wuhan, I felt that same dispassionate interest medics like me are often guilty of – marvelling at the power of disease even while being shocked by the scale of such human tragedy. I remember watching Wuhan get locked down, photos of bodies in the streets, 10,000-bed hospitals thrown up in a matter of days. But like so much in modern life, even the daily images and news from China felt faraway, not real. It was just in a box of light – one that I could simply switch off. And I did.

* * *

A family friend messages me a few days later. A high-powered executive in the financial world who grew up with my wife, Sem often drops us medical questions from time to time about various things. Just as I am finishing the morning ward round, I find that a text is waiting for me on the phone:

"Hello. Should we be worried about this virus?"

I think about my response for a little while. *Should we be worried? How did I answer the same question about Ebola a few years ago?*

I reply: "No more than we should worry about the flu. Just wash your hands on and off the tube :)"

Sem doesn't let me get away with just that. "Are YOU worried?" she asks.

I think about this some more. *AM I worried?* I rattle off a further explainer.

"Only to get on the Piccadilly line, but that's not rational. Flu is still more common and dangerous so far."

Sem is happy with that. We make plans to meet up next week. Another phone call comes in about a young man with an infected heart valve, and then there's a cardiac arrest in another intensive care unit, and coronavirus is pushed entirely from my mind.

* * *

The next day, Sem gives me a quick ring. Her oldest, Emma, has a temperature. It's slightly out of the blue – Sem hasn't rung me about something like this for some time. We go through the usual hoops:

"Any rashes, cough, pain?" I ask.

"No," she answers.

"Eating and drinking and playing normally?" I ask.

"Yeah," she replies.

"Doesn't sound like anything to worry about, Sem, just keep an eye like normal," I say.

"Okay, sure," Sem answers.

At the time I didn't really put those two conversations together, but over the following week Emma's temperature didn't come down. There is no mention of coronavirus, but Sem is in touch far more than normal. Sem's mother has a long-term severe and incredibly complex chronic health condition, under the care of an international super-specialist, and has suffered nearly every complication under the sun in Sem's lifetime. Understandably, Sem is often anxious about health. After two days of fever, Sem takes Emma to the GP, who diagnoses a viral illness. Emma stays well, gets over it, and almost certainly just had a simple cold or viral illness that kids get all the time. But I've got two kids too, and Sem's anxiety affected me in the same way.

Sitting down that weekend, I pull up some of the latest news from Wuhan. Human-to-human transmission, proving that the virus can spread among communities, has been confirmed, and the first smatterings of positive cases in Europe are on the news. Dilsan looks over my shoulder.

"Sem messaged me too. ARE you worried about coronavirus?" she asks. We've gone back and forth on this already, I'm thinking. I try to be completely objective. Wuhan is locked down, the Chinese government is throwing up a 10,000-bed hospital in 10 days, and we in the UK haven't yet had a single confirmed case.

"I suppose this couldn't have happened in a better country – where else could the government lock down hundreds of millions? They're building an entire hospital in 10 days." I shrug. "I don't think we should be worried. Seriously."

Dilsan doesn't say anything, but it's the kind of silence that speaks volumes. She's unconvinced.

"Just make sure you wash your hands," I add.

"Yes, boss."

· · ·

The day after, 31 January, the first two cases of coronavirus in the UK were confirmed and contained at the infectious disease unit at the Royal Victoria Infirmary, Newcastle. Back in my days working at the tropical disease hospital, many of my seniors volunteered to man the Ebola units at the 24/7 special infection containment ward at the Royal Free Hospital in London (the other high-level isolation unit in the country, alongside Newcastle). One of the infectious diseases registrars, Umar, told me about how these special isolation units are set up. Essentially, the patient's bed sits in a clear plastic sealed box, with ports to access and administer care. Surrounding that is a further isolated area to prepare equipment, and both areas sit inside a negative-pressure sealed room (to allow air to flow into the isolation room but not escape from it), with a double antechamber outside to doff and don the protective equipment.

Doctors and nurses work in two-person shifts to look after the isolated patient, in full spacesuit-like personal protective equipment. I saw some of this kit during a drill at an emergency department in central London during the height of the Ebola crisis in Sierra Leone. It was a particularly busy evening in A&E, and the timing of the "drill", at 8 p.m. on a Saturday, was slightly suspicious. Two figures in full protective gear (full-body suits and hoods with visors) marched through the waiting room and into the severe care area we call resuscitation, conducted their isolation protocol and took the simulated patient to another waiting area. Given that this took place during the Ebola crisis, the sight of these fully-kitted figures striding through the hospital induced half the waiting room to promptly stand up and leave without being triaged. I wondered if the same registrars working on the Ebola cases at the Royal Free would be volunteering again for the coronavirus outbreak. For the first time, the bravery of the act of volunteering to staff these special units struck me – a feeling of pride in my colleagues that would come back to me time and time again over the coming months.

• • •

Around this time, in early February 2020, I'd just completed what had turned out to be a long and painful journey through the machine-learning course and was rejected from my first-choice PhD programme. No matter where you are in your career, rejections like these still hurt. Sitting on the tube again, feeling dejected – a combination of free time and pessimism, the cocktail that fuels all social media use – drew me inevitably back to Twitter.

We've just had our third UK case, in Brighton, not far from my hometown of Emsworth on the South Coast. Imagining the densely packed high streets I remember from trips as a child, Brighton seems uncomfortably close to home. I read this news on the way to another of my weekend jobs, a general medicine shift at another central London hospital.

I grab a coffee on the way in, juggling the cup with my phone and my ID badge. I let my feet take me along the familiar route into the ambulatory care area, so I nearly fall over the cordon that now blocks the entrance to the department. A new "Do Not Enter" sign covers the double doors out of the A&E area that I've used a hundred times before. Diverted down several unfamiliar corridors, I eventually find my way back to my room, still, thankfully, on time.

By chance, I know the sister covering the clinic today well. Bernadette is in her mid-forties, a senior sister I've known since my medical rotations as a much more junior doctor. It's easy to get burnt out after a long career in acute medicine, but Bernadette has an infectious energy and sarcastic wit that can make even the worst day seem manageable.

"Bernie," I say, keeping my voice to a conspiratorial whisper.

"Oh, hi Dom. Are you with us today?" she asks. "One day only." I'd tended to start splitting weekend shifts where I could, to get a break before starting the next week. "I'm the special guest today. What's going on down there?" I ask, nodding back to the corridor that's closed at both ends now.

"Oh. They've quarantined it." She nods her head knowingly. "Coronavirus." "Really?" I reply, slightly incredulously, given that cases are still in the single digits. "Well, someone thought it might be. Maybe too jumpy. They are cleaning, anyway," Bernadette answers. Not sure how I feel about this, I go back to my room and pull up the list of patients for the day. It looks busy, but in the end a third of the patients don't turn up.

Bernadette catches me at the end of the day, and I mention the high number of people that didn't turn up. "Expect more of that." Again, she nods her head knowingly, with a glint of a smile in her eyes. "Coronavirus?" I enquire, but I know the answer. "Exactly." She cackles. "I'm just messing with you. It's a Saturday – who's going to want to ruin it by going to the doctor?" "Fair point. Do we know what happened with the corridor patient?" Bernadette shrugs. "No news is good news."

Despite Bernadette's reassurances, A&E looks slightly more empty than normal too. I try to ring some of the missing patients, but only one responds and is happy to receive their blood test results over the phone in any case. But suddenly coronavirus has leapt from my screen to a sort-of reality, even if it is just a scare. It's uncomfortable being immediately so close to it.

My dad feels the same way, as I gather from an email that pops into my inbox that evening. The subject reads "THE DEADLY CORONAVIRUS". For context, my dad was raised Catholic but left Catholicism for the Revelation Church in middle age and remains a committed Christian. He takes a very literal view of the Bible and has written three books on creationist theory, laced with both biblical and geological science. We take quite different approaches to our faith, which has led to some fractious conversations in the past, more so since Dad became interested in the various sinkholes of inter-net conspiracy as well. Despite writing three books that cover planetary formation, Dad now tells me the world is actually flat after all. Such is the power of the internet. All of which is to say, whenever there's a sniff of an apocalypse coming – war in Afghanistan, Ebola, Brexit (!) – my dad will fire off a quick email to remind everyone that the world is ending, and that we should all repent. The DEADLY CORONAVIRUS email carries with it the same tones of loving fatalism and is addressed to the whole family: "This evening we heard of a case in Brighton and I expect it to spread from there to Emsworth [where my dad still lives] in a few days.... The Bible warns us of pestilences such as the Coronavirus as a sign of 'the beginning of sorrows'.... I will need a little while to email a short article about survival in the last days. Love Leander."

Not for the first time, my dad is worried about the world ending, a preoccupation not unique in his generation. I try to stay upbeat in my reply: "Hello dear family, although there has been lots of coverage about coronavirus, so far it has been quite well managed, especially in the UK. We have had three cases to date – the chap in Brighton was travelling from Singapore; he self-isolated and was taken to London, so I wouldn't worry too much. There have certainly been worse epidemics in the past, 1918 for example, and hopefully with modern treatment all will be okay again this time. God bless, Dom."

I phone my dad the next day to reassure him. We chat about work; no, I haven't seen any coronavirus yet, yes, I am washing my hands. Dad seems happy with that. We set a date to visit in a few weeks.

The very next day the papers are vilifying the gentleman from Brighton as a "superspreader", identifying him in the papers. Probably off the back of the email from Dad, the headline infuriates me. This man has every right to his anonymity, and when I dig into it, I discover that he had self-isolated before he even had symptoms. Blaming individual patients, and pillorying them in the headlines, is sensationalist and wrong. The last thing we should be doing is discouraging people from identifying to health professionals that they have suspected coronavirus and hiding them in the community.

I tweet along these lines on one of my commutes to work, a brisk chilly run to the station and then 30 minutes down the Piccadilly line. Swiping through my Twitter feed, something catches my eye. In the replies I find a recurring theme, with people dismissing coronavirus entirely as "just flu" and declaring everything else "media hysteria". Up until that point I haven't really looked hard at the research around the "Wuhan coronavirus". Trying to catch the tube Wi-Fi, I spend the journey trawling the literature, trying to answer the question: *is it worse than everyday annual flu?*

Thinking about my conversation with Sem two days prior, between stops, I read a little more on the "Wuhan" virus. Viruses have a few key characteristics to look at: how they spread, how easily they spread between humans, and how deadly the virus is as a percentage of the cases of people it infects. In terms of how they are spread, both influenza and the "Wuhan coronavirus" appeared to be primarily respiratory viruses, meaning they are transmitted via coughing and sneezing, or touching an infected surface and then touching your mouth or face and transmitting to your nose or throat that way. There were some reports of coronavirus found in faeces as well. It also turns out that normal annual influenza virus is not that infectious, relatively – 10 people might pass it to 13 other people, although it depends on the year. This concept of how many people a single infected person will pass the virus on to is called the R_0. For influenza, the figure is around 1.3, so each carrier will pass on the virus to, on average, 1.3 people. This varies with the properties of the strain that year, so annual influenza is more infectious some years and some years less so.

Coronavirus reports from Wuhan suggest that one person might spread it to between two and six other people, making it twice to nearly six times as infectious as everyday flu. While it is true that annual flu has a high death toll, that's based on the fact that some years' flu variants can infect a large number in a country. Some flu strains cause no symptoms or only very mild symptoms in a high proportion of those infected and are only identified due to the presence of antibodies after the infection has passed. Flu will typically infect between 5 and 10 per cent of an entire population each year. With such a high caseload, although there appear to be a lot of deaths, as a percentage of the number of cases, influenza isn't that deadly in most years, with around 0.1 per cent of those cases dying. This figure is the case fatality rate (CFR).

Coronavirus, on the other hand, appeared to be much more deadly, with reports from China showing that 1–3 per cent of people were dying (10–30 times the rate of normal flu), although it was very unclear how cases were being defined and tested for. If 100 people test positive and 3 diagnosed cases lose their lives, the case fatality rate is 3 per cent. But if the case definition changes, for example because the test is found to be not very accurate (which it would indeed turn out not to be) then we may include as "cases" those diagnosed with suspected coronavirus based on symptoms alone. If the same 3 people die, but this new case definition defines 1,000 people as "positive", then the CFR goes down to 0.3 per cent. This is also heavily reliant on trusting the data being recorded, which there was some doubt about. Trying to work out what might happen to any given individual infected looked increasingly difficult. What *was* evident was the need for large numbers of ventilators (machines that take over the process of breathing) and intensive care beds, which appeared to be needed for around 5–10 per cent of those infected – but again this was all reliant on testing accuracy and reporting.

As I was digesting this information, I came across a report of an outbreak on a cruise ship. The *Diamond Princess* had a passenger disembark in Hong Kong who tested positive for coronavirus on 1 February, and the entire 3,711-passenger ship was then quarantined off the Japanese coast for two weeks. In this closed population, the number of people who died was about 2.3 per cent* of diagnosed cases. Among the infected people, a good proportion had no symptoms, but with so many other factors – including the fact that it was a very unusual and select population, with people in close proximity to each other but also shut into individual rooms early on – all of this had to be taken with large pinches of salt. As I sat flicking by tube stations on the Piccadilly line, I suddenly had the uncomfortable realization that this tube connected directly to Heathrow airport. The same tube I ride back from work every day, along with hundreds of thousands of others. I put my hands tightly in my pockets and tried not to touch anything.

The first big clinical study of patients infected with coronavirus was published at the beginning of February. Out of the

---

* https://www.medrxiv.org/content/10.1101/2020.03.05.20031773v2

138 patients admitted to Zhongnan Hospital in Wuhan, China, 4.3 per cent died. Shortly afterward, on 11 February, the World Health Organization (WHO) announced "COVID-19" as the name of the new disease. COVID-19 got its slightly robotic name to avoid the stigma surrounding some of its epidemic predecessors: Middle East Respiratory Virus, German Measles (not Measles), and Spanish Flu (not Spanish) – the latter being the last comparable pandemic, that of 1918, which I'd mentioned in my email to my dad. It occurred over 100 years ago and resulted in the deaths of an estimated 3 per cent of the world's population. The R_0 was around 1.8, and case fatality may have been as high as 10 per cent. And this took place in a world before planes, trains and automobiles – a world far less connected than today.

I changed tubes and looked up other coronaviruses, wondering how we managed SARS back then. By comparison, it seemed that COVID-19 could spread easily without symptoms, while SARS patients were usually feverish when they were infectious, making them easy to isolate and quarantine. COVID-19 could also last on surfaces; one paper I found suggested it could live on metal, glass and plastic for up to nine days* and still infect a person. So we were dealing with a virus that easily spread, was 20 times more deadly than flu, was harder to detect in people and could cling to surfaces all around us. My hands dug deeper into my pockets, and, when I got off the tube, I picked up some hand sanitizer at the chemist.

. . .

* https://www.journalofhospitalinfection.com/article/S0195-6701(20)300 46-3/fulltext

The next few days were a sea change for me. My ears would prick up when I heard any mention of COVID-19. On my commutes and breaks I continued to hoover up studies and news. Twitter became a valuable resource of other doctors and experts sharing and debating the research. Among the obligatory memes and outrage, Twitter emerged as the world's largest medical forum. The topic: SARS-CoV-2 (the virus), or COVID-19 (the disease). Through all these sources, the numbers I'd only just started to pay attention to painted a bleak picture. A picture I'd seen before.

A few years ago, a web developer worked with a group of virologists and epidemiologists to create a pandemic simulator. The mobile game was called Plague Inc. and the premise is relatively simple: with limited resources you craft an infection of various qualities (air spread, water spread, etc.) and choose where in the world to start it off. As the game progresses you can evolve the infection, with the ultimate aim of infecting the whole world and wiping humanity out. It's hard to contemplate anything so alien to us as exponential growth, but this was a great way of relaying the concept. The only way to successfully win was to create a virus that spread easily, didn't cause many symptoms initially and had a lowish mortality rate, meaning it could spread further before measures were taken against it. Early quarantine measures in a country was always a game-ender for the virus. And here was COVID-19, in Plague Inc. terms, following the same winning formula. The game became so popular it spun off into a board game called Pandemic, the sole goal being the destruction of humanity. In the same way that we enjoy disaster movies and apocalyptic conspiracy theories, we seem to have an inherent fascination with our own downfall.

The numbers from the studies in China, at least, were inescapable. They revealed a long infectious period, a long subsequent illness, many asymptomatic or only very mildly symptomatic patients spreading it around and a clear predilection for the elderly and those with comorbid conditions (i.e. those with another disease or condition). At least initially, all reports indicated that children were nearly entirely spared. That evening, sitting in the nursing chair with my son sleepily settling in my arms, I remember thanking God for that at least.

· · ·

By genuine coincidence, I'd asked Dilsan to keep a lookout for a Bible. While I've never been particularly religious, the rest of my family is far more so than me, and there are parts of Christianity I don't understand or agree with, which is often a point of division. In one of my flurry of ideas, I thought it might be good to get hold of a Bible and actually read some of it, if anything to bring me closer to my dad and brother than to God. By the time we got around to finding a Bible, a leather-bound Gideon, rescued from a charity shop, it was the middle of February and reading it took on a different quality.

Increasingly, the news and social media seemed more worrying and hectic. My phone felt hot and caustic in my hand by the end of the day, and the cool leather of the Bible felt like a balm. I started to read the New Testament each night in small segments. I found it calming and familiar, and having to concentrate to follow the text helped me switch off from everything else. I told my dad about it the next weekend over Skype. He started crying. There was no less division, but at least we had more to talk about.

* * *

That weekend I had taken on some extra shifts again, this time covering two peripheral hospitals, which I needed to drive between. Both sites had ward rounds to do and new patients to see – it was tough work to get everything done in the morning and get to the next site to start over in the afternoon. One of the patients was a young young woman named Gillian. In her mid-twenties, Gillian had never unwell a day in her life, had just got married, and ran her own company. For the last week Gillian had felt sore in her chest, particularly at night time. When the pain had started to worry her, particularly on the left side, her partner had brought her into A&E.

The blood markers (a sign of a disease or condition observed in a blood sample) suggested there was some damage to the heart muscle, and the medical team suspected a myocarditis – inflammation of the heart muscle. As this usually follows a viral illness, the unit staff had put Gillian into a side room. Outside her room were a stack of thick, white medical-grade FFP3* masks, the standard precautions at the time for seeing a patient with a possible respiratory infection. We put gloves on, and one or two fell on the floor and were discarded. Being slightly over-vigorous as I detached the plastic gown from the dispenser roll, it tore and had to be binned. At the time, we as a profession would sometimes dispose of unused PPE for very little or no

---

* FFP standing for Filtering Facepiece Respirator, with the "3" denoting the highest of the three classes of filtering efficiency

reason – there never seemed to be a shortage. Finally ready, myself and the SHO in the ward, Kate, entered Gillian's room.

Gillian looked well, sat up in bed in her normal clothes. I introduced myself and Kate, our voices slightly muffled through the thick masks. I asked her the routine questions for a patient with suspected heart problems. Did she smoke, or drink, or use recreational drugs? Any family history of heart disease? No, no, no, no, came the answers. I asked the last routine question – Have you had any cough or nasal symptoms lately? – something we ask as most myocarditis cases in young people occur after a common cold or similar.

"Yes, actually, I had some sniffles about two weeks ago. Slept it off."

We wrote that down dutifully. I looked hard at the ECG and asked, "Does it hurt more when you lie flat?"

Gillian nodded.

"What about when I press here?" I asked, gently prodding over her ribs.

Gillian shook her head.

The electrical tracing of his heart remained stubbornly normal. I explained things to Gillian.

"Okay. It looks like the heart muscle and the outer lining of the heart have become inflamed. This is called perimyocarditis. This usually happens after a cold virus or similar. We will keep you in and monitor your heart rhythm and blood markers. Most cases will get better by themselves and, once we see that, we can let you go home." Another patch in my "cloak" from a previous boss, I always finish explaining a diagnosis with, "What are your questions?"

The first one Gillian asks is: "I don't have coronavirus, do I?"

It's the first time I've really had to think about it in the real world. There have been some case reports of COVID-19 causing inflammation of the heart coming out of China. Kate and I exchange looks over the top of our masks.

"Have you travelled at all recently?"

Gillian shook her head.

"Have you met anyone unwell that had?"

Again, a head shake.

"Then there's no reason to worry," I tried to reassure her. "This is all just precautionary – let's get your bloods checked tomorrow and if they are improving and everything else looks okay, we can get you home on Monday, after a heart scan."

Gillian thanked us and we shuffled out.

Once out of earshot and writing up the notes, Kate paused when she came to the part where Gillian had asked about coronavirus.

"Um. What shall I write about this?" she asked.

To be honest, I had no idea. The testing criteria were still only for those with symptomatic illness and a travel history that included Asia. I wondered at what point we would start screening these viral patients for coronavirus routinely. We'd just had a further five or six people diagnosed in the UK, but the numbers remained minuscule, so it seemed ridiculous then to even talk about it. Equally, coronavirus could be a very mild illness and those small number of cases were only the tip of the iceberg of an already established community epidemic. I deferred the decision.

"Can we ask microbiology what they think?" I asked. Kate shrugged and added a note to her list of jobs.

I removed my mask and I went to throw it away. Changing my mind at the last moment, I stuffed it in my pocket instead, in case I'd need it later, as we used to do during flu seasons when I worked in general medicine.

We rolled the computer on to the next patient.

The next day I came back in the afternoon to catch up with Kate. We'd seen so many more sick patients, including two that we'd sent to the tertiary heart hospital, and, after an even longer shift at the second site, I'd completely forgotten about Gillian. As we rattled through the list, Kate reported that Gillian's blood markers appeared to be getting better, having fallen from 420 to 310 (the convention in myocarditis is that once the levels of troponin – a protein released into the bloodstream when the heart muscle is injured – start to fall consistently, the patient is safe to go home). Overly cautious, I suggested we keep her in to make sure they continued to fall the next day as well.

"Oh yeah. What did micro* say?" I asked.

Kate gave me a half smile. "They were quite nice actually, said it was an interesting question, but they can only test for the criteria as they are at the moment. Only for travellers."

"Fair enough," I answered.

"Caused quite a fuss with the ward nurses though," she added.

"Oh. Shit. Sorry. Well, at least we asked the question."

We moved on through the list.

· · ·

---

* Slang for the microbiology team

Somehow the FFP3 mask has made it into my bag and lodged there for the weekend. I wonder how long they actually last for, and in retrospect probably should have thrown it away long before, but I couldn't bring myself to do it. That Monday morning, I stand on the tube platform with my mask stuffed in my jacket pocket. A few other commuters are dotted along the chilly platform. I stand there, hesitantly waiting for the tube and wondering if I should wear the mask.

As the tube pulls into the station, I bottle it and keep it in my pocket. Finding a seat in the corner, I sit down and get my laptop out. Loading up one of the coding exercises, I glance up. A young couple sitting opposite are both wearing disposable surgical masks. It's an occasional and not unusual sight around London, one I've often scoffed at in the past, but now seems increasingly sensible. Still feeling too self-conscious, I leave the mask off, but spend some time looking at the evidence for masks and coronavirus. All I can find are papers about flu, which indicate that wearing a mask reduces infection by four times compared to no mask at all. Somewhat buoyed by this couple and the evidence presented, I wear the thick damask mask on the commute home. Jostling among hundreds of commuters in a packed tube carriage, no one so much as bats an eyelid. This is of course London, and only the most extreme indiscretions on public transport will break the unwritten rule of no eye contact or acknowledgement what-soever. It is slightly hot but actually quite comfortable. I try not to touch anything and use hand sanitizer when I change stations. Feeling foolish for ever having felt self-conscious in the first place, I tell Dilsan about it.

"Interesting. Do you think it really helps?" she replies.

"Not sure, but it stops me touching my face at least." I am a well-recognized self-face-toucher.

"Maybe Ehsan should wear one too."

My brother-in-law had a liver transplant as a child and has been on immunosuppressant medication ever since. For a number of reasons, this group in particular appear to be more vulnerable to the virus. The next day I message Nes about getting some masks, and give them to Nes to pass on, advising Ehsan to avoid public transport as much as he can and wash his hands assiduously.

In the midst of this, Nesli and Ehsan are looking to move house. We'd tried unsuccessfully to live together for a while, but four kids in a single household was too much work for any one person. Several houses in the area are for sale, but they're pricey for what they were, even for London. Pressures on school places has inflated prices higher still. We spend a few weekends looking over houses for them, including a place on our street, although it seems suspiciously cheap. After some digging, we find that it has no freehold and is quite run down. The year Dilsan had spent on maternity leave, no longer just around the corner from Nesli and Ehsan, had been particularly hard on her and the kids, and we're keen, if possible, to try and recreate the close distance we had had in Tottenham once more. It makes a nice break from obsessing over COVID-19 to trawl through Zoopla or similar and look at properties. Just out of interest, I take to working out what we could buy together if both families escaped from London to somewhere sensible. I find a seven-bedroom house a hundred miles from Leeds, with its own stable and outhouse and 20 acres of land that we could afford for the same price as two two-bed houses in Tottenham.

My own sister, Beck, a singer-songwriter, was also in London, and her career looked to be on the verge of exploding. She was gigging nearly weekly, dropped her first track onto Spotify under her artist name, LEIO, and had picked up interest from the upper echelons of her industry. One rainy Tuesday on a day off, we meet up for an impromptu coffee. I try to give her the big-brotherly and much-needed life advice that I'd given her before, and she dutifully ignores it. If it were up to me, she would quit her current job working 60 hours a week at a high-end spin studio, find a higher-paid, lower-hours job, focus on her music, and save rent by moving into our attic. She, of course, refuses. She is also completely unconcerned about coronavirus, to the point that I think maybe I shouldn't worry so much either. It's hard to convince her otherwise, despite the numbers or the evidence, and she just thinks it's hysteria. She's so upfront about it and reasonable that I can see myself in her eyes. Maybe I am being hysterical, I wonder. I shrug, we finish our coffee, I show her Dad's email, she rolls her eyes and then she has to dash off to a recording session.

I catch up on some life admin as the sun goes down, and then go and make an extremely rare appearance at the pub to meet some old friends. When I originally moved up from the quiet South Coast to go to medical school in London, many of my friends and family took a pretty dim view, Mum especially. She'd banned me from applying to more than one medical school in London and would have much preferred that I went to Southampton and lived at home. Needless to say, I didn't apply to Southampton. In fact, I changed my medical school choice on a whim on the day of the UCAS application from Imperial to UCL, the only university that actually accepted me and the place where I met my wife. So much of our lives hinge on such seemingly small decisions.

In my first year a friend of mine from school came up to visit, arriving at King's Cross at 5 p.m. on a Friday. A particularly busy rush hour, every entrance and exit was packed shoulder-to-shoulder with thousands and thousands of commuters squeezing through the catacombs of the underground. Waiting outside the station, I could just make out Laurence's very red face and tousled blond hair as he waded upstream against the river of people, a massive rucksack strapped behind him. When he eventually broke free of the mob, he seemed happy to see me, but visibly shaken.

"I've never actually seen that many people before," he told me.

It's easy to forget how densely packed London is compared to the rest of the UK. Over time, several of the circle I grew up with moved to London, and several of the more sensible ones moved back home again too, especially when they got round to having kids. Once in a blue moon, when all the stars align and I'm not working, those of us still based in the city try to meet up. Keeping in touch with people who you've known your entire life is a good way to stay sane, especially as life overtakes you.

By the time I get to the restaurant, Rob and Tom are already there, and, grinning like a Cheshire cat, is another childhood friend (who is supposed to be in Sydney and has flown in as a surprise), Jonny. The food is great, the wine is better. Eventually the talk turns to COVID-19 when Jonny announces he's heading to Singapore the week coming.

"I wouldn't do that." I'm slightly glib, probably having had too much red wine, but I'm genuinely worried. Jonny is unperturbed.

"I'll be fine, it's only the older people that need to worry," he says. I shrug. That's certainly what the studies were showing. "We still don't know that much about it, and even if only 1 per cent of young patients get really sick, that could be you," I warn. "You aren't really convincing me here, Dom," Jonny answers. "Look, if you can avoid travelling I really would. Also, you could be fine, but others might not be." "Mmmm." Jonny thinks about it. He, of course, goes to Singapore anyway.

When I get home, slightly tipsy, Dilsan and I catch up. My sister isn't worried, Jonny isn't worried. Maybe we shouldn't be overly concerned after all. In a clumsy way, I try to make the same compelling arguments I've heard that day, how coronavirus is only a real risk to the elderly and it'll just be like a slightly more severe flu season, but I can't make them land with the same confidence. Dilsan is unconvinced.

"Maybe. Let's hope so, I guess."

• • •

Later that week, after 10 days of continuous working, I'm feeling pretty burnt out. Dilsan has had a shit day and, our moods compounded by the biting cold and seemingly perpetual dark, we sit sullenly together over bowls of soup. She slides her phone across the kitchen counter.

"It's in Italy now."

On 22 February, the news reports a major outbreak of nearly 80 cases in northern Italy. Eighty cases in a cluster, a cluster only a few hours away by plane, feels like an explosion, a distant earthquake. Unlike China, Italy's media and social channels are open to us, and already we can feel the tremors in our timelines. What was once the "Wuhan virus" became COVID-19 and is now in a major European country, heading toward a significant outbreak. There had been reports in Singapore and South Korea, but an outbreak in Italy feels like a huge and frightening leap toward us. For the first time I ask the question that keeps coming back. The question that sweeps all the assurances away again: "If it can happen in Italy, why not here?" A knot of anxiety twists in my chest.

CHAPTER 3

Incubation

Over the coming days, cases double in Italy every two days, and while there is general unconcern in the wider world, Twitter is aflame with testimonials from Italian doctors and nurses, increasingly concerned by the ferocity and volume of cases. It seems that Italy is headed for a severe and large-scale outbreak, given that around 23 per cent of the population is over 65 (compared to approximately 19 per cent in the UK). Yet, while the Italian patients are older, their wealthy and well-resourced healthcare system has twice the critical care beds we do, with 12.9 critical care beds per 100,000 people to our 6.2, and 3.99 doctors per 1,000 people to our 2.85.*†

Letters, photos and videos from Italian colleagues fill my news feed and fuel my nightmares. They read like dispatches from a not-too-distant battlefield, a modern-day Western Front. One account is piercing, describing intensive care units being overwhelmed in days, with makeshift units overtaken just

---

* https://stats.oecd.org/Index.aspx?ThemeTreeId=9#; https://www.politico.eu/article/charting-europes-capacity-to-deal-with-the-coronavirus-crisis

† https://stats.oecd.org/Index.aspx?ThemeTreeId=9#

as quickly. It sounds like pandemonium, with unwell patients over 65 reportedly not even being assessed for intensive care, and doctors who haven't touched a patient in decades being yanked out of labs and backroom offices and thrust into the field, clutching onto nothing but some written instructions for using the most basic breathing support machines and a prayer. It feels like so many of our colleagues in Lombardy* are screaming, but somehow the message doesn't penetrate the wider consensus, like they're in a padded room, locked away and muffled. Maybe I could partly have understood this if we had been talking about China – respiratory viral outbreaks like SARS and MERS were part and parcel of the region in many minds. But I couldn't remember any of the relatively recent epidemics breaking out like coronavirus was doing in Europe.

But despite the gravity of the situation in Italy, it appears as if here we are carrying on as usual. Flights from Lombardy to the UK, as with every other country, are still taking off every day, without quarantine or tracking when they landed. The government are insistent we would take measures at the "right time", to avoid fatiguing the population, but I couldn't understand why we weren't taking the most basic precautions right now: disinfecting transit hubs, providing hand sanitizer and advising the public to avoid areas of infection and to self-isolate if returning from areas where the outbreak had already taken hold. Even more baffling to me was the constant proclamation that our healthcare system was "ready" for coronavirus.

---

* At this point, the "epicentre" of the outbreak in Italy

After having spent the best part of the last decade writing about, campaigning for and studying NHS capacity and resources, the suggestion that we had the "capacity" to cope where Italy made no sense. We already had 100,000 missing staff, £6 billion in infrastructure debt and the worst waiting times for A&E, operations and cancer targets since records began. Not to mention nearly the lowest number of nurses, doctors and hospital beds per capita, especially intensive care beds, in Europe. In one ear came the stories from Italy, a well-provisioned healthcare system completely overrun, and in the other came the narrative from the UK, that the NHS would be fine without any special provision or preparation, despite all evidence to the contrary.

A light of hope in a tunnel of darkness, Dilsan passes her driving test at the end of February. Suddenly free, she wants to drive everywhere, so we take the opportunity, with Ayla deposited at nursery, to sneak off for a morning date with the baby. Over breakfast, we try to work out how all these moving pieces won't end up the exact same way as, or even worse than, they had in Italy. I idly doodle on a Costa napkin as we sit sipping coffee in the window seat. Zach sleeps blissfully in his buggy next to us. The winter sun dances between us. Dilsan pulls the napkin from me.

"Let's just do the numbers. How many intensive care beds do we have?" she asks.

"About 3,500," I answer.

"And how many do we think will be infected as things stand?"

"Well, Prof Whitty reported the worst-case scenario as 80 per cent of the population. So 55 million or so."

"And how many will need an intensive care bed?"

"Well, supposedly 5 per cent of those, so around 2.5 million."

"Okay, well that's rubbish. What about if it's only limited to 10 per cent of the population?"

"That's about 6 million people, so 300,000 people needing critical care, and if the case fatality is actually 1–2 per cent then that will be 60–120,000 deaths, assuming everyone gets an intensive care bed that needs one, which isn't possible."

Dilsan chews the top of her pen nervously.

"Well, what about if only 1 per cent of the population are infected?"

"So 600,000 people infected, 30,000 will need intensive care. That's still 10 times what we have right now."

"These numbers don't add up."

"Nope."

Dilsan is looking really shaken, and so am I.

"What can we do?" she asks.

I'm desperate to reassure her, but I don't know what can be done. Dilsan's dad lives in Turkey, bordering another major outbreak in Iran. He has sent us literature about the measures the Turkish government are putting into place, including disinfecting transit hubs, installing thermal cameras at airports and at borders, and producing and providing masks for the public. My own Aunty Joyce in Berlin has told me that Germany plans to lock down the whole country to fight the virus. With mass testing and six times the intensive care beds than us, Germany seems to be taking measures we aren't. It appears we are doing nothing, and I can't understand why.

· · ·

Later that day, I feel awful. My head is pounding, my throat burns and I feel congested. I've lost all energy, have no appetite and get a sudden bout of diarrhoea. I put it down to overdoing it, too many weekends back to back, or maybe a spot of food poisoning. I soldier on like this for a day or so, but by the next day I feel like I can't do anything. Dilsan sends me to bed. Usually I can't sleep during the day, but I crawl into bed sniffing and fall almost instantly asleep. I sleep for most of that day and into the morning of the next, and wake up feeling nearly completely normal. The following day, I'm back at work.

* * *

A few years ago I was working as a medical registrar at one of the busiest hospitals in the country, in what was then the worst winter crisis in the NHS on record. (Every year since then has been statistically worse.) While the snow tipped down outside, it settled on a line of ambulances queuing into the A&E. This scene of cold quiet belied the chaos inside.

On a normal day we might admit 20 medical patients to the hospital, but today we admit 60 – all desperately sick, all in need of more than the five minutes my team can give them. The referrals telephone rings incessantly, and my emergency pager bleeps so much it develops its own staccato rhythm. For every bleep I can answer, two more will go off while I'm on the phone. I try to buy lunch on the way to a referral, pay and then have to sprint to a cardiac arrest call. It's two hours before I can pick it up, and I eat it trudging back to A&E. It isn't medicine: it's firefighting.

On top of the torrent coming into the hospital, no one has seen the clinical decision unit patients, 10 patients from the previous day waiting for a medical team to review and manage them. It isn't clear who is supposed to be looking after them, so it has fallen on the medical dogsbody – the medical registrar on call, me. I whip around and make quick decisions to keep everyone safe until tomorrow, when I hope there will be space and time to do this properly. I get the feeling every day is like this here. The day is littered with makeshift solutions to the litany of problems: there's no ambulance to transfer a patient urgently to the heart centre – I have to call three times and go and meet the ambulance crew to navigate the queue outside; and there's no second registrar, so we divert a senior SHO to hold the emergency pager while I take the complex patients. All the bits I really need time to do properly, there isn't time for.

A terminally ill mother of three comes in close to death. There's no bed on the ward and we can just about find a side room in A&E to give her some privacy. I have to break the news to her family in a linen cupboard alcove, the quietest place I can find. I finish the day feeling physically beaten; the night team goes through the list, and the names and stories seem endless. The next day is exactly the same.

Over three years, things had only gone in one direction in the NHS – A&E waiting times in England had hit an all-time low and continued to dive; targets for performance were broken so many times they were scrapped; a picture of a sick child on an A&E floor had become a political lightning rod just a few months prior, but fizzled out again without any consequence. And now, as COVID-19 tore through the better-resourced Italian healthcare system, overwhelming patients and staff, with daily reports of medical colleagues losing their lives, each news briefing bravely trumpeted that the NHS was "ready" for COVID-19. "Ready" despite having the fewest beds, staff and resources of any modern healthcare system in the world. "Ready" despite the ballooning waiting lists for people needing cancer surgeries and those in crippling pain from arthritis needing joint replacements. "Ready" despite no radical measures being put in place to increase ventilator capacity and personal protective equipment stocks, to rapidly train staff or to protect vulnerable areas such as care homes. The numbers were inescapable: the caseloads were rising. It felt as if we were sleepwalking into disaster. I genuinely felt like I may become hysterical, I was so desperate to find some objective evidence of why we shouldn't be acting now, shouldn't be at least doing some mass training, but I couldn't find any. Every conversation I had with friends or family or even colleagues ended in the same half-shrug of the shoulders, with no option but to "trust" it would be okay. The word jarred because, as doctors, we are always taught that "trust" simply isn't good enough. Plan for the worst and hope for the best. But we were only doing the latter. All the while we could physically *see* our own future coming down the line, just two weeks ahead of us in Italy. It was obvious then that global pandemic was inevitable, and yet we weren't reacting.

That evening I wrote some of these thoughts down, at first as a thought experiment. Later, I developed it into an article covering the scale of the potential need for intensive care and PPE, the high burden of deaths, the lack of current

NHS capacity and the major issues with those non-coronavirus patients who would not get looked after for every COVID patient that came in.*

It's almost difficult to imagine what it was like writing down the numbers that we had been talking about in the abstract for weeks prior. Tens of thousands in intensive care, thousands of deaths, and that was the most conservative estimate. Where local healthcare had been overwhelmed, in northern Italy and parts of Iran and even in Wuhan, the mortality rate was much higher than 1 per cent. Spelled out like this, it looked disastrous. I wasn't sure whether publishing this article was a good idea or not. The UK government was spending a lot of time and effort trying not to induce panic about COVID-19, claiming that aggressive measures too soon would "fatigue" the population. I took a different view; I work with the public all the time on the worst days of their lives, when they are really sick and their lives or those of their loved ones are threatened. In my experience, with the proper information and rationale, which it is my job to provide, people have a nearly limitless capacity to adapt and to rise to the occasion, whether for themselves or their family members. As for following advice, once we are clear and transparent on the risks and realities of medical advice, most people recognize what the right and sensible thing to do is, and do just that.

For example, the absolute best time to convince someone to stop smoking is before they ever start. But if you can't do that, the second-best time to convince them is immediately after they suffer their first heart attack. For many patients in

---

* https://www.huffingtonpost.co.uk/entry/nhs-coronavirus_uk_5e58e642
c5b6beedb4e98eb9

modern-day society, a major heart problem is the first time they have been severely unwell in their lives; even a minor scare with chest pain can force people to confront the reality of life and their health with wide and sober eyes. But, universally, what people need to help guide their life choices is trusted and clear information, a particular well that has run nearly dry in our present society, with a deluge of misinformation in newspapers and social media to contend with. What never works is making decisions on behalf of people, without rationale or transparency or shared decision-making. Abrupt discussions, without giving people an opportunity to be heard, makes them feel like they're being steamrollered, or just not looked after. It's natural for some to resist that. We have to respect the autonomy and capability of the people we look after – it's not our job to make decisions for them, but it is our duty to make sure they are fully informed of the benefits and consequences of those decisions.

The article I wrote would be seen as inflammatory and scare-mongering, and would have personal and professional repercussions, but I honestly said nothing that hadn't been said already, just a clear and transparent spelling out of the titanic scale of the pandemic to come, especially if we were to do nothing at all to prevent it. It's been bandied about so much that the term "public duty" in the medical world is almost already a cliché, but Dilsan and I both felt the pull to act on those grounds alone. But deeper than that, I was trying to protect not just ourselves, but Ehsan, my dad and our colleagues in hospitals who would be bearing the brunt of the onslaught on the frontlines.

I sent the article in, and it was published the next day, on 28 February, and I went to work like any other day. The title came out slightly more provocatively than I'd intended, but the body of the text stood as intended. The wavefront of the virus had jumped from Wuhan and Singapore to Tenerife and Italy, and had now reached our front garden – now was the time to sound the alarm, because time was all we had then to prepare. Time we weren't using.

That day I was on the rota to attend the cardiac CT scanner, a relatively new piece of equipment that can look at the heart arteries with a traditional CT scanner in super-quick time. We sit at the back of the scanner while patient after patient is brought through, performing the vital checks to make sure that what is being indicated on the display is correct and that all of the medications we give to slow the heart and dilate the arteries will be safe for the patient. We give high volumes of these medicines to each patient and scan perhaps as many as 30 patients in a day, so there is a substantial amount of prep to do to get hundreds of medicine vials drawn up ready for use to make sure we can still report the scans and do all the other tasks during the day.

I arrive early when only the cardiac radiographer is there, Mark, who helps me get the drugs out, and I plonk myself down to work through the hundred or so vials in front of me. For these sessions I'm often paired with a colleague, which makes it somewhat more sociable than some of the more isolating activities, like clinic. As I'm robotically twisting off the glass vials and drawing them up into labelled syringes, my colleague for the day comes in; today, it's Hugo.

I highly respect Hugo; a few years my senior, he's a really sharp guy with a brain the size of a planet and someone who genuinely cares about things, whether that's research or colleagues or work – he speaks with a passion about everything from football to psychology. Our kids are similar ages and he has already given me key advice about going into a PhD, as he is just coming out of one. He also loves a good argument, the cut and thrust, in the way that some academics will naturally want to debate with an intensity completely unrelated to the topic, just for the joy of the process. We chat a little as Hugo sits next to me and we make a mini-factory line, him opening the vials and me carefully drawing each one up. It's monotonous work. Naturally the conversation turns to COVID-19. I ping Hugo my article. He reads the title, "The NHS isn't ready for coronavirus".

"So what healthcare system *would* be ready for a pandemic?" It's a fair question for him to ask, but deliberately simple.

"Well, we could be a lot more ready, and that's the point," I say.

"So how many ICU beds would we need?" Hugo asks.

"Tens of thousands in the worst-case scenario there," I reply.

"So how would we possibly find those beds?" he answers.

"Well, I doubt we'll be able to find all of them," I admit.

"So how could we be 'ready'?" Hugo replies. I get his point.

"I suppose the answer is twofold: 1) Anything we do right now, even if insufficient, is more than we started with, and will save at least some lives. 2) If we could never be ready, our only solution is to suppress the virus for as hard and as long as possible, to at least buy the time to do 1), if not await a vaccine."

"There is no vaccine. It would take years."

"Perhaps. On a normal scale. But everyone in the world will be working on the same problem – the normal rules won't apply."

"This is just speculative. We will cope as well as any other country. Will France do any better than us?"

"Probably – but better to speculate on the worst and be transparent about the risks. Why are all the medical conferences being cancelled, when public mass gatherings are still going on?"

"This remains to be seen. You are not an expert here."

"I don't pretend to be. I'm just a guy with Google and a napkin. I would just really like someone to show me where I've got this wrong."

"We will have major incident plans and cancel leave, and we will adapt and cope."

"Would it be nice to have more time to adapt, though?"

"Fair enough."

"Time will tell, I suppose."

"Indeed."

What I really respect about Hugo is that he's really happy to let an argument get heated and then completely defuse it.

"Come on, let's go and get a coffee and I'll tell you about this great idea I have for a book about lobsters," he says.

Grateful for the exit, I give a nervous laugh, partly because I don't think he is actually joking.

. . .

That same day I get home to find Dilsan watching the news. I make a quick plate in the kitchen and come and sit next to her on the couch. She's watching BBC News 24, which we never watch. Every story is coronavirus-themed now. The headline of the day is: "First community transmission reported in the

UK". Someone has been diagnosed for the first time in the country without any link to the epidemics in other parts of the world. Unless we very quickly hear reports of a further two or three cases, those other patients are now lost in the community, as are their subsequent contacts, and the contacts of those contacts. The invisible enemy has now been set loose among us. COVID-19 has landed. Dilsan rests her head on my shoulder and we watch the news unroll quietly.

CHAPTER 4

Symptoms

The next morning, 29 February, I wake up with the kids and let Dilsan sleep in. We are trying to get Zach on solids, and I've never seen a baby eat like he does. From day one he's been on three full solid meals a day. Feeding him is like trying to shovel coal into a steam engine – he can clean an adult-sized plate in three minutes. Ayla is her own little lady now, sitting on the counter, criticizing my breakfast service until I give in and we make pancakes like she wanted in the first place. With both kids happy and settled in their chairs, the sun just breaching the horizon and some gentle Bill Withers (Ayla's favourite) crooning on the wireless speaker, it feels like another world. Ayla is smearing Nutella industriously over her second pancake and I feed a bit to Zach, who's never had chocolate before. He makes a "mmmmm" noise and Ayla nearly falls off her stool with laughter.

When we were first pregnant with Ayla, all our friends and family told us how tired we would be, how much we would love them, how it would completely transform our life priorities. But what no one tells you about kids is how hilarious they are. Whatever else is going on in the world, they don't care or know about it, and their joy is limitless and untouched. It's energizing, and as I lean on the counter, making Ayla laugh as I put marmalade on her pancakes like Dad used to do for me, I feel myself reset. This is what is truly important, and we work backward from there.

Dilsan comes down sleepily at 9 a.m. Both of us are deflated and stretched after last night's news coverage. I think we are both starting to sleep badly, even on nights when Zach sleeps well, which are few and far between.

"Morning!" I say, encouragingly.

I thrust a coffee into her hand and try to get the right balance of lemon and sugar on her pancake. As many married couples will know, putting condiments on each other's food is a high-risk business. It goes down well.

"You seem chirpy this morning?" Dilsan looks at me oddly. I feel good, though.

"Why not? The sun is shining. There's pancakes!"

"And Nutella," Ayla adds, covered in a fair amount of it.

"I'm gonna go for a run. Is that okay?" I ask.

Dilsan is always pushing me to do more exercise, which as a cardiologist I'm guilty of not doing nearly enough of. Pancakes don't help massively either, but the rare weekends no one is working are special occasions in my mind and don't count. She smiles and waves her hand.

"Off you go, then."

I nip upstairs and try to find some running gear. Like all of us, I've gone through fits and starts of exercise, joining gyms and then letting my memberships languish, so my wardrobe of sportswear comes in phases, and I try to find something that fits. Throwing on some bits, I launch downstairs and stick my headphones on.

"Get some milk!" Dilsan shouts to my back as I jog out the door, playlist already pumping.

The morning air is crisp and my breath huffs in front of my face as I jog off down the hill to the local park. Like a clunky car engine, parts take a while to warm up and get moving, but I feel I have boundless energy and charge headlong into the park along my usual route. I don't notice the little traffic cones and the slight crowds around as I charge on, and it's not until I spot one or two attendants in hi-vis jackets that I realize I've just gatecrashed a fun run. Trapped on the route now, runners ahead of and behind me, I'm routed around the park on a far longer route than I would normally take. By the end I'm puffed out, being far less fit than I'd hoped. Resolving to do that more regularly, I hobble slowly down to the shop on the way home again.

Outside the little Tesco, the papers are displayed. The first headline, in one of the less salubrious tabloids, is "Find the hidden carriers!", which kills my jubilant mood. There are several milestones toward adulthood, but realizing the tabloids are utterly useless as sources of actual facts and news is one of them. I read on, infuriated already by the tone of the front page. "The race is on to find the contacts of the first community transmission case of coronavirus," it begins. I wonder why they're still reporting this – it's too late. As soon as they have found a single infected person without a connection to a travelling individual, that means the virus is spreading invisibly in the community. If the virus has an R_0 of 3 (the likely number at the time), that means there are already 2 other people infected plus the original patient. In a very short time, around 6 days, those 3 cases will become 9 cases, and then 27 cases, and then nearly 100 cases. This has already been going on for a while. Understanding exponential increases is completely alien to the human mind – our mammalian brains are set up to follow the linear path of a problem from A to B to C. We can't readily leap from A to D to H.

The best analogy I have come across to date is trying to imagine a small space, perhaps your childhood bedroom. Roughly 2 x 2 m perhaps, so 4 m squared. What would it look like if it doubled every day? On Monday, you can just about fit a child's bed in there. On Tuesday, it's the size of the living room, 4 x 4 m, or 16 m squared, so you can get in a full-size couch set and TV and still have space for an armchair and a coffee table, and a kitchen-dining room. On Wednesday, your bedroom is now 64 m squared, the average floor space of an entire house. By Thursday, your bedroom is the size of a doubles tennis court, and by Friday, a football pitch. By the next Monday, your childhood bedroom is the size of a London borough, and by the Monday after that, larger than the entire planet. The only way to see realistically into next week is to plot the numbers like this, point by point, with cases doubling roughly every two days. By this rough estimate, Italy looked to be nearly exactly two weeks ahead, and by this point in full meltdown in Lombardy already.

There are now two obvious and inescapable truths – that the virus can no longer be contained, because we aren't testing or finding contacts anymore, and that without widespread measures it will continue to double every two to three days. And yet still nothing changes. It occurs to me then, puffing in my running gear and looking at the collective journalism of our country spread before me, that a global pandemic is now inevitable. At least the tone of the conversation has changed – there is some realization of the scale of this disaster – but it is no less ill-thought through. The next tabloid reads "Govt will call up retired medics to fight coronavirus". A group of men and women in a high-risk group, coming back to a service they've only just, I can only assume happily, retired from. The article is light on details – where will this Dad's Army come from? How will they be deployed? How will they be monitored and professionally regulated? Feeling slightly worse for wear now, I buy the milk and trudge back home. The buzz of the morning rush is receding fast, dropping me into a grim mood.

When I get back, Zach is down for his nap and Ayla is holding a dinosaur/teddy bear conference on a table in the living room. A blissful moment of peace, I make Dilsan and myself coffees and we sit and listen to Ayla hilariously narrate this important meeting next door. It's mostly about "not sharing". Curled in the corner of the couch, Dilsan's eyes are slightly red, and she is huddled in a blanket, sitting hunched over her cup. She must see my concern.

"Feel a bit rough this morning," she says. I press my head to her forehead. She doesn't feel warm. "Think I've got that tummy thing that you had a few days ago." We get the thermometer out anyway, but she doesn't have a temperature. It's the end of winter, and there are hundreds of all the usual chest and tummy bugs out there still, and she has no cough or fever or any of the other typical COVID-19 symptoms. I make her some tea and send her to bed for the rest of the day.

Dilsan emerges for dinner only, and then goes back to bed again. She finds it hard to eat anything, either. With everybody asleep, I sit in front of the laptop trying to work on a grant proposal. I can't help but be distracted, as if by a scab I cannot stop worrying about, and I find myself diving back into the COVID-19 papers from Wuhan. We've both had a strange diarrhoeal illness which sounds viral, with muscle pain and extreme fatigue. It's in the small print but there it is: around 10 per cent of patients with coronavirus experienced abdominal symptoms, of pain and diarrhoea. Although mostly presenting in children, it has been seen in adults, too.

I feel completely fine. None of us has had any fever or cough, just a vague headache and congestion. Am I being completely paranoid now? Should I go to work? I check the government guidelines carefully – the only symptoms they talk about are cough and fever. We have had neither so far. My internal monologue is broken by a cry from upstairs: Zach has woken up. We can't seem to crack his sleep and he has good nights but many bad ones. A 9 p.m. wake-up is an omen of a bad night ahead.

I go upstairs to pick him up and settle him. He always does the same thing when I get him: puts his head instantly on my left shoulder and straightens his arm as he tries to rush to sleep on my chest. I listen to his breathing gently settle as the music from his star-light chimes. He sounds a little snuffly. Does he feel hot? While he still sleeps, I try to manoeuvre down the stairs again and, one-handed, find the contactless thermometer. It makes a little beep pointing at his forehead, which Zach snuffles at while remaining steadfastly asleep. It's 37.2. Normal. Relieved, I pop back upstairs and gently lie him down. His breathing is congested but he is settled. Does he have COVID-19? Do I? Every day it seems we know less and less about it. I creep into bed next to Dilsan and listen to the quiet of a whole house asleep, but the thought is like a penny in a jar, rattling in my head all night.

I didn't sleep at all that night. It was the first of many nights like this.

* * *

Dilsan lets me lie in the next morning, but at 7.30 a.m. I am woken by Ayla's raised voice. Every toddler has the odd tantrum but it's unusual for her to be so vocal in the morning. Groggily, I trudge downstairs. I share a look with Dilsan. "She's really grumpy this morning," Dilsan says.

She looks a bit red around the ears. Despite her protestations, I trick her into taking her own temperature. She presses the little button and it pings – it's 38.2. Ayla has a fever. I feel my brain physically splitting into two. Cool-rational-doctor Dad brain assesses her like I have a hundred times before – any rashes, lumps or bumps, tummy pain? She's drinking fine and peeing, and I can't find anything else wrong. She doesn't even have a cough, maybe just a slightly drippy nose. Meanwhile, paranoid-about-COVID Dad brain is overheating already, trying to recall incidences of childhood hospitalization and symptom frequency, and establishing where the nearest A&E is and if we know anyone working there. I know this is likely just the kind of viral illness kids get up to 20 times in a winter, but that's my rational brain talking.

Dilsan is more sensible. She gets some Calpol and Ayla drinks it down and settles to watch "Hey Duggee" on TV.

"It's probably nothing," she says, but she gives my hand a squeeze anyway. "What about work?"

That's a good point. I have to check the latest guidelines. NHS staff are only self-isolating for contact with known cases, not for household fevers, at least not yet. So back to work we will go. We keep Ayla out of nursery and ensure that she's topped up with Calpol. She seems a little tired and grumpy, but there aren't any other symptoms. I sit with her watching television, surreptitiously timing her breathing, Googling the normal breathing rate for a three-year-old. It's quite an effort to wrench myself out of this cycle. We try to keep the day as normal as possible, but we are walking on eggshells the whole time, snapping at each other, hardly saying a word in between. The stress of worry, without being able to do anything, is like a hot white wire stretched taut between us. Naturally, the kids are oblivious, and we look after them like any other day. It gets us through, to be honest. Ayla seems no better, no worse, and goes to sleep early. Zach is sniffly but settles. I feel like I've run a marathon when we collapse onto the sofa that night. Dilsan is already flicking through a research paper about COVID-19 in children, writing the odd note on a pad beside her.

"I think we should put our phones away," I announce.

There seems to be some resistance, but something gives. We put everything away, turn the TV on, and try to find a slice of normality.

The following day, my parents are scheduled for a visit. Dad is over 80 with chronic lung disease. My mum is 20 years his junior, and generally fit and well, but she looks after my gran, who is 85 and still lives at home but needs a lot of support. Ayla's fever still comes and goes, and neither me nor Dilsan feel quite right yet. My sister Beck is supposed to come round as well. Having endured a very rough week herself, she's really looking forward to it. I've bought a shoulder of lamb, my specialty, and it's ready to roast. Then, Beck calls me around 8 a.m. – she hasn't been feeling well and has a chronic cough and headache, but no fever. She has some bloody mucous coming up. She isn't worried (and still wants to come over), but I am.

Equally, I haven't seen Mum and Dad since January and neither has Beck. Ayla, feeling better this morning, is jumping off the couch in excitement that Grandma and "Grandma-Dad" are coming over. I yo-yo between paranoia and clinical concern. As ever, when we try to exercise medical judgement when one of our family is involved, it falls to the opposite partner to be the final arbiter of sense. Dilsan lays it out:

"Your dad is very high-risk, from the kids and possibly from Beck. It probably isn't COVID but do you want to risk it?"

I don't. It's a little heartbreaking. Mum takes it in her stride, although I can hear the hurt in her voice. Beck understands, but she is really upset. So we Skype Mum and Dad instead. We chat about religion and Dad is more engaged over the webcam than ever. I reflect on how lucky we are to have this technology, which even just a few years ago was not capable of enabling a human interaction like it can do now.

I can't get hold of Beck for the rest of the day, and when we finally catch up, she's crushingly disappointed. Her living arrangements have chopped and changed so much recently that our house has become a sanctuary for her, a port in the storm. I try and convince her to come and stay for a bit longer when she's better, and she's grateful but declines, as ever. We set a date with Mum and Dad to come up again in two weeks' time, but privately, I doubt this will actually happen.

Just as we are finding common ground with Beck again, our brother from the US messages, asking, "Does Beck have coronavirus?" Unhelpfully, it transpires that Dad got the wrong end of the stick and sent a classic family email to everyone to tell them Beck has COVID. I spend the rest of the next day trying to unwind this, still wondering if we did the right thing by cancelling.

· · ·

Tuesday 3 March falls on the date of a pre-booked study course – as part of our training we have to sit a comprehensive cardiol-ogy exam covering every aspect of heart diseases. It's textbooks' worth of material to cover, but there is an annual course organ-ized by colleagues from the US-based Mayo Clinic that blis-ters through the content. It cost my entire year's study budget, which I will have to claim back, but I've heard good things. It isn't clear if it'll be going ahead – despite the government guidance to continue with mass gatherings like conferences, many colleagues around the world have been systematically cancelling the usual gatherings of medical colleagues. There is a clear chasm between the approach of medical professionals and the national policy itself, which I can't explain. Ayla is still unwell but seems a little better than yesterday. Not going to the conference will mean losing the upfront cost I've already paid on a credit card, money we can't afford to lose. A mass gathering, with very senior and esteemed colleagues from all over the world, seems like a bad idea, though. Dilsan and I decide together that I should go, so as not to lose the money more than anything, while taking some precautions.

This time, I make the journey wearing my mask, religiously avoid touching anything on the tube and wash my hands vigorously with my pocket hand sanitizer at every opportunity. It's already half-empty. The coffee shops are no longer taking reusable cups, the first time I've noticed businesses adapting to COVID-19. No one else is wearing masks. I get to the conference hall early, find a seat at the back well away from anyone else, and hunch over my laptop. At some point I sneeze and feel incredibly self-conscious. The audience is entirely cardiologists, from my level up to some of the most senior professors in the world. Oddly, no one is taking any specific precautions. COVID-19 gets a mention in the opener, but only as a tongue-in-cheek joke. There are some polite titters in the audience. No one appears concerned. During the breaks we all gather together and share coffee and network, and I even meet one or two personal heroes of cardiology. We stand super close – there is no social distancing or even mention of it. Life seems to be carrying on as usual.

At the conference, I bump into another registrar from my deanery, a really pleasant surprise. Nat has nearly finished her training, having lengthened it to have her two kids. She's super competent and one of those people that exudes positive energy. She looks worried when we start chatting, though.

"So how worried do you think we should be about coronavirus?" Nat asks.

"I think it's going to be a total disaster," I say, too glibly.

Nat looks crestfallen.

"I'm so anxious about my kids," she says.

"It doesn't really affect kids seriously at all, Nat, thank God," I caveat. "At least not in the studies so far."

"At all?!" Nat asks. "I need to look at this."

"Ayla's got a fever right now." I sigh. "I'm still worried about it."

"Are you wearing a mask on the tube?"

I sheepishly show her my mask.

"Aren't you self-conscious?" she asks.

"You get used to it," I tell her.

"Mmmm."

I send her the papers I've been looking at and our conversation drifts to other topics. At some point the session recommences and we file in again. I begin to wonder, with anxiety at home and so few of my peers doing similar things, have we gone mad? Are we hysterical? I try to focus on the rest of the day. I realize that I've really missed lectures – my muscle memory of holding a pen and scribbling on a clean notepad transports me to younger, freer days. I focus, and forget everything else, just for a little while.

. . .

On the way home, I text Dilsan about her day. Worried about Ayla's fever, she cancelled on a birthday party that Ayla was supposed to go to. When she phoned to let our friend Jas know, it turned out she had already decided to cancel anyway. Jas was an anaesthetist and then a GP. She sends me a photo of another mutual medic friend of ours wearing a mask, who has been doing so since February. Many other professionals seem to be thinking along the same lines.

"Did you see this, by the way?" she messages. It's a story about how my favourite beer, Corona, is going out of business in the US because some people think it's related to or even the source of coronavirus. I am saddened by how unsurprised I am by this.

I flick through my Facebook feed. There's a message from my Aunty Mo. She's a retired nurse, and on family gatherings we would always find time to seek each other out and chat about some aspect of work. She has some great stories. Her message reads: "Saw your article on Coronavirus. Agree wholeheartedly! Word on the grapevine is Jeanne's John thinks it will be serious. Stay safe!" This sends a shiver down my spine. Jeanne is my cousin, and her husband is Professor John Edmunds OBE, infectious diseases epidemiology professor at the London School of Hygiene & Tropical Medicine and a preeminent member of the Scientific Advisory Group for Emergencies (SAGE) that is advising the UK government on their COVID-19 response. The decision-making the government refers to as being "guided by the science" comes from this large and voluntary group of scientists. John was one of the foremost response planners to Ebola and was awarded the OBE for his modelling work in controlling the epidemic in Sierra Leone. He is a brilliant, compassionate and decent man. Although it is a distant third-hand opinion, if he is that worried about this virus, then perhaps we are all vindicated in worrying too.

· · ·

The next day, the conference takes on a different tone to me – it seems wasteful, ignorant even. I grab one of the aisle chairs well apart from anyone else. I wonder if they'll cancel it before the end of the week. Two major cardiology conferences have been cancelled already.

Meanwhile, Ayla is getting better, and at home the waters appear more settled, while abroad something feels like it's brewing. I've become obsessed with the daily rises in COVID-19 cases – the web pages tracking Italy and the UK have become fixtures in my phone. The reports from Italy across social media are so frequent, graphic and surreal that it's hard to read them at all. The numbers are indisputable – with cases now in the thousands, Italy's deaths have just reached over 100. Our own figures are tracking theirs to the day – doubling every 2 or 3 days, we are nearing 100 cases already. Italy went into national lockdown at 322 cases, so the benchmark for how we may respond is only 4–6 days away.

I find it hard to concentrate that day. I'm grumpy and distractible – there's just so much misinformation out there. Scrolling through my timeline I find several repeated tropes: "Coronavirus is just flu", "Antibacterial washes don't work", "It's all a hoax". Trying to do something constructive with all of the social media time, I spend an hour or so on the tube trying to put together a short explainer on COVID-19 for the general population. I call it "Everything you need to know about Coronavirus. A thread by a doctor".

What we know about coronavirus at this time is based on limited information from Wuhan for the most part, and some early indications of what is happening in Italy. Although the typical symptoms of fever and cough are relatively common, muscle pain, loss of appetite and pain in the abdomen and diarrhoea occur in only a small fraction of cases. Loss of smell and taste as a common symptom has emerged as well. Most people, around 4 in 5 of those infected, will have mild symptoms, and perhaps as many as 1 in 5 will have no symptoms at all. Up to 1 in 5 will be incredibly unwell and require intensive care. Overall, between 1 and 3 in every 100 cases will lose their lives, which varies significantly with age, with case fatality rates up to 15 per cent in the over-eighties. In Italy, the overall case fatality rate was looking close to 10 per cent, which may reflect the inability of the local healthcare system to cope.

As viruses go, this one is particularly stealthy, with a long incubation period (thought to be between 3 and 24 days at the time, but since recorded as around 7 days) during which time it can be passed on to others by people who aren't themselves experiencing any symptoms. The best intervention remains washing your hands, which has the double effect of avoiding you accidentally touching a contaminated surface and then touching your face, as well as of preventing you from spreading the virus via your hands to other surfaces or people and infecting others. Some viruses (like norovirus, the winter vomiting bug) can't be removed by alcohol hand-sanitizer alone, but coronavirus definitely can, which makes a big difference when you're dealing with a virus that is 3 times more infectious and 10–20 times more deadly than influenza, not to mention the fact that coronavirus also has no vaccine and currently no definitive antiviral treatment, unlike influenza.

Unlike other coronaviruses, like SARS, where infected patients are nearly always feverish, with COVID-19 a much higher proportion (up to 50 per cent) of contagious patients have no temperature at all, making them much harder to quarantine, for example in airports. Despite knowing how infectious it is, and having multiple confirmed locally transmitted cases at this point, we still aren't testing non-travellers in hospitals, even if they have suspicious clinical symptoms and signs, like the patchy pattern of pneumonia we see on CT scans of the lungs. Professor Whitty has stated that, unchecked, the virus could infect up to 80 per cent of the population, putting huge strains on beds, staff and resources. The only defence against the virus at this moment is the strict public health measures of hand washing, avoiding unnecessary travel and working together. This is the ultimate challenge to the post-truth selfishness. A pandemic requires trust, transparency and common decency, so we all should be informed, be kind and stay safe.

I never know what will and will not make an impact on Twitter. Often I'll feel there's a vital gap of something unsaid that I will spend hours researching and crafting a piece to fill, only to find that just a handful of people are interested. Similarly, I can dash off a few lines about my cat and make the national news. (This is a true, and incredibly weird, story.*) Nevertheless, the short explainer, in which I present simple facts about COVID-19 as if I were talking to you as a patient, takes off on Twitter, and a journalist from the Press Association gets in touch. They want to record a video version of the text

* https://www.dailymail.co.uk/news/article-6499273/Cat-rescued-spending-hour-stuck-engine-bay.html

for online media. I haven't really done anything out loud or to camera before; it's really not something I would consider a strong suit of mine. Dilsan is on the fence about it. In the end, I slightly reluctantly agree to do it the next day.

The following day at the conference there are noticeably more empty seats and a slightly thinned crowd at coffee time. I wonder if colleagues are staying home voluntarily, perhaps those who can afford to lose their fee better than I can. The event centre lets me use the members' area at lunchtime and a very nice cameraman from PA called Steve spends a rather awkward 40 minutes getting me to read out the threads and taking some pictures. I'm really uncomfortable and I plan not to do this again. Toward the end of the day, I find out that I have an on-call shift that evening, so slip away early to get across town in time for handover at 5 p.m.

After a few days away from the hospital, it's actually quite nice to go in – it's easy to get worn down by the rigmarole of early finishes and late starts, but a few days' rest and the love-hate relationship rebalances. I suppose the warning signs will be when it doesn't. I pop up in the lift and roam around the ward to find the day team. There's only one patient coming in that evening, a young woman arriving for assessment about whether she might need heart surgery, and everyone else seems settled for now. I take the emergency pager and phone from the day registrar, check in with the junior on the ward, and then sit down to review the notes of the patient coming in.

As I'm doing so, one of the consultant infectious disease doctors, Dr Chiltern, comes into the office to sit at the station next to mine to update some documentation, on his last case of the day. James was the senior registrar when I worked at the tropical disease hospital, and we have worked together on projects in the past. Over the years we've bumped into each other fairly regularly at lots of workplaces, London hospital medicine being a relatively small world, especially within the deaneries. One nurse I've worked with, Nick, was training on the cardiac ward when I was first starting as a registrar at that hospital, and moved within a few weeks of me to my next rotation at a completely different hospital, before he left that job only for me to start working with him again the next year at the tertiary heart hospital (where we still work). These strands of connection become more and more common throughout our careers.

Anyone who knows Dr Chiltern is immediately struck by two qualities of his: firstly, exceptional brilliance, and secondly, exceptional affability. Everybody has their own professional demeanour, but the friendly and calm energy of James has always been a joy to work with. I recently contacted him about my idea to try to analyze the natural menagerie of bacteria in poo and its link with, and potential treatment for, obesity using artificial intelligence. We start chatting about that project here. Despite being incredibly busy and it being well after 5 p.m., James seems enthused about the idea and in great detail, goes into the specifics of how it might work. He gives me a few contacts and finishes up his documenting. Getting ready to go, I trouble him with one more question.

"Are you worried about coronavirus?"

Caught on the hoof, James gives it some genuine thought.

"I suppose," he says, pausing, before adding, "Not as worried as I should be."

It strikes me as such a strange thing to say, but such an honest one. Perhaps it's what we should all be saying. The concept of cognitive dissonance, believing two contradictory things simultaneously, is simply a part of being human. We spend far too much time trying to justify our thinking, to make it logical like the ordered world we try to create, but we aren't consistent or rational beings, and our brains are not simply mushy circuit boards. This cognitive dissonance, of understanding the huge potential scale of coronavirus and yet simply not translating that into true concern, seems nearly universal. It's an attitude I encounter over and over again, an attitude that comes and goes even in myself, born from a desire to not think the unthinkable, to reject how surreal our actual reality is about to become.

I mention this conversation to Dilsan, and she just laughs.

"Wait till you get a load of this," she says.

She loads up her Facebook and opens some of the medical groups she belongs to.

The same conversation is going on over and over again; some medical professionals seem more worried, some are completely blasé, and many are somewhere in between, managing to accept both the scale and impact of the epidemic, but also holding the belief that normality will prevail. Like one obstetrics registrar, who wonders if she will need to cancel her holiday to Italy in two weeks' time, while also understanding that cases in Italy are doubling every three days and that they are about to lock down entirely. There's also an intensive care consultant admonishing another intensive care consultant for claiming "It won't be that bad", without being able to produce a shred of evidence to justify that assessment. Likewise, some GPs are planning to close their surgeries, while others mention planning to open additional services that same month. It reads like a boiling sea of conflicting ideas.

One prevailing theme is the touchstone of the Chief Medical Officer. As a group, we don't particularly trust politicians, wearing the scars from too many past battles, namely contract disputes, policy fights, pay freezes and union and funding scuffles. But generally, doctors are driven by evidence, and will listen to one of their own, or at least give some semblance of listening. What's so strange here is that so many conversations descend into the same shouting match, coming down to the same point: "Don't you trust Prof Whitty? Don't you think they know what they're doing?" It's a common viewpoint, but such an alien one in the world of medicine. When we look at new therapies or medicines, we scrutinize the published research meticulously, not who publishes it, but the data they present. We trust opinions, but in a court of law "Dr Smith told me to do it" is not a valid or sufficient defence. And we also know, as a collective group of scientists and clinicians, that there is a large committee of people trying to process a body of imperfect science and statistical estimates and squeeze that through a political filter. What was unique here, like in a war or other society-changing event, was that it seemed to be pushing us to abandon our natural inclination to evaluate and scrutinize and to plump instead for blind trust, something we would never normally do. Questioning the advice, rather than being seen as the healthy scientific debate our entire way of life is built upon, often became labelled as "scaremongering" or "undermining" that trust, even in closed, clinician-only groups like those on Facebook.

Like every other section of society, the doctors were human, and their opinions, like everyone else's, seemed to span the entire spectrum from bunker-building preparation to outraged scepticism. What disturbed me was how shallow the sceptical end of the pool of conversation was. I had convinced myself we were heading into historic disaster but was so desperately looking for something tangible to suggest the opposite. The facts coming from Italy, however, remained immutable, despite the reassurances of the UK government's nightly briefings. Reality was bearing down on us, but we didn't want to look. I closed the laptop in frustration. I could understand the confusion and division, but what was the government doing? The guidelines hadn't changed, community transmission was established, and yet there were no measures to stop the spread, even ones that required no energy or input from the public.

The next morning, the Prime Minister, Boris Johnson, was on "This Morning", discussing coronavirus. The clip was edited, but one of the strategies he mentioned was to "take it on the chin" and let the virus pass through the population all in one go. In more formal terms, Sir Patrick Vallance, the Chief Scientific Adviser, had discussed the rationale behind making early interventions in a similar way, introducing the concept of producing "herd immunity". Herd immunity is normally a concept we talk about with vaccines – it means if the majority of people (the herd) are vaccinated against an infectious illness, even if not every single member is, the illness finds it impossible to spread and will be effectively stamped out. Think of it as a "sea" where the illness cannot go, which surrounds each member that is still vulnerable. The "herd" as a whole is immune from infection, even if some individuals are not. It takes a high number of immune individuals – somewhere around 80 per cent of the population – to create herd immunity.

There are quite a few immediately obvious problems with this as a strategy for coronavirus:

1) There is currently no vaccine. That leaves only natural infection to create herd immunity, whereby the population would "take it on the chin".
2) There isn't much strong evidence that being infected with coronavirus actually produces protective immunity, although it is likely.
3) Given the statistics about COVID-19's spectrum of illness, with up to 15 per cent needing intensive care, and as many as 1–3 per cent dying, infecting 80 per cent of a population of 66 million people would lead to millions requiring intensive care, and millions of deaths.

All of this is reliant on NHS capacity to cope with cases. As soon as that is exceeded, other people who develop potentially life-threatening conditions other than coronavirus will also die where they otherwise wouldn't have.

Everyone in the health service is acutely aware that there is very little spare capacity in the system for additional work, and that anything we do will have to be at the expense of something else. On the face of it, pursuing herd immunity as detailed above seems like a horrific, even insane, idea. But I wonder if there is perhaps a middle way, a way in which the most vulnerable can be protected while the herd produces sufficient immunity to weather the virus and not overwhelm healthcare services in the process. Experts like Sir Patrick Vallance begin to expand upon this sort of approach, talking about "flattening the curve" – spreading the number of new cases over sufficient time that NHS healthcare resources wouldn't be overwhelmed to the point of collapse, and allowing some viral spread to create an exit plan.

I wonder, if we attempt to "flatten the curve", how flat does that curve have to be to stay under NHS capacity? The numbers of ventilators, anaesthetic consultants and intensive care beds and staff are readily available to Google, so on the tube, I do some back-of-an-envelope maths, factoring in 80 per cent of the population being infected, and work out how many cases a day that would need to be to stay under the red line of maximum NHS capacity. Being as generous as I can, I still find that we would need to nearly triple the current capacity in order to flatten that number of cases below it. Like trying to fill Wembley Stadium through a single turnstile, what would the length of that queue be? Even if there were two or three turnstiles? To achieve herd immunity through natural infection and stay within that capacity, the pandemic would take over 10 years to manage, and that's excluding the work we would shift capacity from. We cannot ignore cancer and heart operations for a decade.

This clearly was not a viable strategy. A vaccine would be the only other means to an end, and the only way out. Yes, we were unlikely to develop a significant vaccine within a year, but the options appeared to be impossible vs. unlikely, so a choice of no choice at all. What other information there was, economic consequences and modelling data, for example, wasn't in the public eye. From what was available, this was the scenario.

What potential consequence the government had modelled for locking down much earlier I'm not aware of, but when faced with either 10 years of a flattened curve, or 12–18 months awaiting a vaccine, a week's difference would have no impact on the ability of the public to cope with the measures. But with cases doubling every two to three days, a week would mean a four- to eight-fold difference in the number of those infected. I don't believe that when faced with dire emergencies the public gets "fatigued". Was the Blitz boring? This paternalistic approach lacked transparency and vastly underestimated the British public's resilience, the same resilience I had witnessed for eight years in some of my patients' darkest hours.

The strategy was essentially immune to logical evaluation: its lack of transparency made it inscrutable. You either had to trust the strategy was correct, or you didn't. But if you didn't, every day meant an exponential step closer to utter disaster. On the face of the testimonials from Italy and the numbers from all over the world, it simply didn't make sense.

· · ·

That weekend (7/8 March), I am back on-call, meaning another safari between hospitals. The morning starts early. The tubes are thankfully empty. I put my hands deep in my pockets and keep my mask on up to the top of the escalators. It's a cold day, and taking the mask off becomes a shenanigan as the straps catch in my headphones and tug my hat off. I go into a packed coffee shop, where it's hard to keep any distance from anyone. I get a coffee and nip across the road, just in time to get to the office in the acute medical unit before 8 a.m. The cardiology rounds always start here, seeing the new patients the medical team have admitted overnight with heart-related problems. It's only been two weeks since my last on-call shift, but the hospital is noticeably different. There's a soft electric tension in the air, like a coiled spring. About to go off.

The boss is Dr Bream, a genteel heart-failure specialist, who is incredibly accomplished given he's only a few years into his consultant career. We know each other enough to say hello, and as we make our slow way round the usual suspects of cardiology complaints, we chat about each of the cases. A gentleman in his nineties with a pacemaker has collapsed at home. We ask to get his pacemaker checked to see if there are any dangerous heart rhythms. Conscious of the impending epidemic and the risk posed to the elderly with pre-existing conditions, I ask gently if we should consider getting the pacemaker check done urgently so this man can go home. Dr Bream wrinkles his nose at the suggestion, and he is right of course, it isn't a justified request in normal times with such limited resources. But these aren't normal times. Dr Bream remains unconvinced. We move on.

I'm looking at each patient through a new filter now, asking myself if they *really* need to be in hospital. Might they be safer at home if the ward fills up soon? I see a 40-year-old very fit man with a minor rise in his blood test markers after a run and some back pain that sounds like a muscular problem. There's also a 60-year-old lady with a known irregular heart rate, which is still running slightly fast, but without any symptoms. She stays in to slow her heart down a little more. Keeping these people in are typical procedures in the "safety first" style of defensive medicine we have been practising for a long time. But I can't stop wondering if we're doing the right thing. Even so, I don't suggest any more novel discharge solutions and we finish the round promptly at 11 a.m.

Dr Bream heads off to another hospital, and I tidy up the list of patients before getting ready to go to a different hospital. The medical team is chatting in the office, and I stop by to fill the juniors in about the heart patients we've seen, updating them on any jobs, scans or bloods that need organizing, and to check in to see if there are any other referrals to see before leaving. The team is looking at a particularly awful chest X-ray, which looks like a dense fluffy white butterfly when it should be a clean dark one. The lungs are filled top to bottom with patchy fluid.

Being nosy, I ask, "What's going on there?"

The junior doctor on the ward, Mark, shrugs. "Young guy from 'the take'* a few nights ago. A&E had him down as heart failure."

I look back at the chest X-ray. It doesn't look much like heart failure to me; in fact, it doesn't look like anything I've seen before. I must make a face when I think this, because Mark catches it.

"Yes, exactly. Steve was the registrar on, asked three questions and then left the room. He phoned the patient on their mobile and did the rest of the consultation from outside."

"Coronavirus?" I ask.

---

* "The take" is the term we use for the patients freshly admitted to hospital from the A&E department

"Well, that's what Steve thought. We couldn't test him because he hadn't travelled anywhere," Mark tells me.

"It's a community disease though now, right?" I ask.

"Guidelines haven't changed, though. Lab just bins them if we try to send them. Need microbiology to approve. Only sent to them yesterday."

At that moment, a senior acute medicine consultant sweeps in. Her badge reads Dr Farrukh – I've not met her before.

"Okay, we will need a medical reg for tonight. Any takers?" she says.

Apart from me, already on call for the weekend, everyone else in the office is still very junior. This seems to occur to Dr Farrukh as well. "Were any of you on with Steve this week? You'll need to self-isolate if so," she says.

Mark and I share a look. Mark pipes up. "Is this about this chap?" He prods the patient details at the top of the X-ray screen in front of him.

Slightly surprised, Dr Farrukh eyes the X-ray and nods.

"He was positive then?" Mark asks.

"Yes, the lab just called. First swab came back positive. What's the story?" Dr Farrukh asks.

Mark fills her in with what he knows so far. She's impressed that Steve had thought on his feet, outside the guidance. It's the first real-world case of confirmed coronavirus I've seen, even tangentially.

"How's the patient?" Mark asks.

"In ICU. Second case here now." Dr Farrukh hesitates for a moment, and then her phone goes off and she has to head out again.

"Oh, God," Mark says. He's reading back through his patient's notes. "I just remembered, he's a train guard."

I stare at the X-ray and catch the blood tests as Mark goes through them again. Some of the blood counts are unusually low, namely the blood-clotting red cells (platelets) and the infection-fighting white cells (lymphocytes). We Google some of the typical features of COVID and find a carbon copy of the X-ray. Once we see it, it's impossible to unsee. In fact, there's another patient on Mark's list with identical blood results. A young woman from east London, with a cough and a fever, but no travel history and no "risk factors" for coronavirus. We pull up her X-ray: it's not as florid but is strikingly similar. She's in a side room and they've sent flu swabs, but haven't done one for coronavirus yet.

"She's got coronavirus." I say. At least until proven otherwise.

Mark is sceptical. "She hasn't travelled anywhere," he says.

"Neither had your patient in the ICU. It's a community disease, and has been for over a week now." I reply.

"Why would we get two in such quick succession?" Mark asks.

"Well, let's see. You've had two cases in the last three days, so you should expect to have four cases today. Eight by Tuesday," I answer.

It's actually really hard to imagine what eight patients with a single illness on even a large ward would look like. It's something that simply doesn't happen, with rare exceptions like the heart attack unit we have at the tertiary hospital. I pull up the Google sheet I've been messing around with, inputting the numbers from the coronavirus briefings and crudely trying to scale them to make predictions. So far the numbers have risen 30–40 per cent every single day. The first patient in the UK died two days before, on 5 March – the same day that Professor Whitty announced that it was necessary to move from the "contain" stage of the response plan to the "delay" stage. I show Mark the predictions. If there were 206 cases nationally today, there would be 400 by Tuesday, and, by the following Monday, over 1,000. We scrolled down to the end of the month, where my crude spreadsheet was predicting over 100,000.

Mark has gone pale. "I'll get her tested," he says, very quietly.

· · ·

It's Saturday 7 March, and it's been over a day since the UK government started routinely testing hospital patients, beginning with intensive care patients. The first results are expected that afternoon. I get off the tube in the weak winter sun, the chilly wind nipping at any exposed part. I've got used to the mask now; it feels almost cosy, especially in the biting cold. The Saturday street market outside the tube station is busy and crowds haggle for everything from saris to roasting nuts to mattresses. Normal life continues unabated.

I cross over and head into the hospital, navigate the complex lift system with slightly more ease than the first time I visited and get to the top floor to the cardiology ward. I chew on a sandwich I grabbed *en route* as I look through the emails to read about the patients on this ward. A general heart ward, the patients here have routine problems you'd find in any district hospital, and usually a fair number of patients without any heart problems at all. Despite specializing in heart medicine,

I have always enjoyed general or "internal" hospital medicine. It's easy to get lost in a niche topic sometimes and forget why we trained as doctors in the first place. The best specialists are always the best "generalists" as well; there's no point fixing a heart attack and missing a lung cancer, or putting in a pacemaker and missing the epilepsy diagnosis. Humans don't come presented in neat parts; as much as I'd like to ignore everything north of the collarbones and south of the solar plexus, I don't get to choose my patients. And they don't get to choose their doctor – a doctor that only looks at their heart, and misses their early kidney failure, might be the only doctor that they get to see.

The first patient on my round is Krish, an incredibly sprightly 80-year-old former shopkeeper. Despite being as bright as a button, three heart attacks in three decades have left his heart muscle barely pumping in his chest, working at just a fraction of the strength of a normal heart. His heart function is kept going with a "whole box of tablets", as he puts it, twice a day. Periodically, something will tip his precarious heart the wrong way, and his lungs and legs will fill rapidly with fluid. His daughter suspects he occasionally stops taking his pills in protest. Now ballooned with 20 kg of extra fluid, Krish staggered into A&E, having taken the bus, with very low oxygen levels. He's on a drip, and slowly getting better, but it's become a daily difficulty to navigate both his heart and a new problem: poor kidneys. I pull the computer-on-wheels into his side room.

"Morning," I say, forgetting it's already well past lunchtime.

"AFTERNOON!" Krish cackles.

His daughter gives me an apologetic smile.

"Apologies. Still going on the morning ward round!" I joke. "Started five miles away."

I press a thumb into his legs, and it leaves an indent 2 cm deep, like pushing into well-kneaded dough. It tells me there's still plenty of fluid. I place my stethoscope on his chest to listen to his heart, and then ask him to lean forward. His daughter jumps up to help but Krish "tsks" and pushes himself up. I listen to the bases of his lungs – I can't hear any fluid. I'm close enough to see the flecks of lunch in his scraggly grey beard. I give a quick feel of his tummy; there's some fluid in there too. His neck pulsates with each beat of his heart.

"Mmm," I say. Still a long way to go, I'm thinking.

"How's it looking?" asks Krish. "Can I go home today?"

I check his weight chart – his "dry weight", the weight he normally sits at, is 65 kg. His weight this morning is 78 kg. We normally say 1 kg a day of fluid is about the right amount to lose with the drip he's on at the moment, so he's nearly two weeks away from being back to normal. With a frail heart and struggling kidneys, and at 80 years old, two weeks is a substantial amount of the likely life he has left, I think to myself. Sometimes we can get people home to come back for a drip for the same treatment, but we would need to manage too many systems for Krish to do that safely. Even with coronavirus on the horizon, the hospital is still the safer place for him.

"It's going to be a while longer, I'm afraid, until all this fluid is off again. A week at least." If we manage a bit more each day, he might get home by then. Krish nods sadly but understands.

"Thank you, doctor," he says.

"Thank you," his daughter says, with a slightly different inflection, but I get her meaning. I feel like this is a conversation they've had a number of times already.

The next patient is Cassie. A schoolteacher in her early thirties, this is not a routine story at all, and I take a deeper dive through her notes from her admission. The top line reads, "presenting complaint" (the term we use for what symptoms the patient presents with): chest pain and breathlessness. Further down, there's a note mentioning "possible heart attack". Cassie became unwell a week ago, finding it hard at first to get the shopping in from the car, and then simply to walk around her house, without finding it profoundly hard to catch her breath. Her partner drove her into our A&E just last night. Her bloods are slightly concerning: one blood marker for infection is slightly low, another is significantly high. Her heart damage markers are increased as well. Not in the range I'd typically see a heart attack in, but well above normal. Her chest X-ray looks slightly hazy, with a subtle triangle of grey on the left that could indicate a lobe full of pus. This looks like pneumonia to me, so far.

I pop into her room, where a lady in an unfamiliar hospital uniform is sitting by her bedside. Both Cassie and her visitor have mousy brown, short hair, olive skin and wide green eyes. Slightly different noses and mouths, of a similar age.

"Morning, I'm Dom, one of the doctors. How are you?"

"Yup, all good." Cassie is sat up in the hospital bed, chatting away, although two tubes jut prominently from each nostril, snaked to an oxygen pipe in the wall. Her eyes are bright, but curls of hair are plastered to her forehead.

"Okay, off you go home, then." I joke. Doctor jokes are like dad jokes – if you were ever to come on a round with me, you'd be sick of mine by patient number three. Cassie and her visitor, I'm guessing her sister, give a little chuckle. "How's the breathing?" I ask.

Cassie takes an experimental breath, and winces slightly on the left side.

"Painful?" It's the same side as the triangle on her X-ray. "Can I have a listen?" I ask.

I take her pulse and it's racing slightly for her age; her slender wrists are warm and flushed. She feels hot at her neck, too. I didn't see much about a fever in the notes, but I'm not surprised. It's common for a temperature to come and go. I put my stethoscope on her back – her heart skips and pounds along and sounds completely normal, but her lungs sound worse than her X-ray looked, with crackles on both sides of her chest.

I check her temperature charts – she has had small fevers throughout the night, but never touching the red line of 38°C, just skulking beneath, with 37.6, 37.8. I used to have an infectious disease boss who insisted that the correct definition of a fever was 37.8°C, and gave an hour-long lecture on the exact reason why, the entire contents of which I have entirely forgotten except for that figure of a supposedly "true" fever. I check her medication chart – despite the diagnosis on my notes of possible heart attack, somebody has already given her antibiotics as well. I spot something else on her chart.

"You take immunosuppressants?" I enquire. Her sister "tsks" loudly. I hate to give the impression I don't know my patient, but this is the first time we've met and there was nothing mentioned about any immunosuppressants in her history on the system.

Cassie isn't perturbed by the question – she rattles off the answer she must have given a hundred thousand times before. "I had a liver problem when I was six. Had to have a transplant. Been fine since but take those pills every day."

Slightly pissed off at myself and the handover for not mentioning anything, I have to start again. Immunosuppressed, nasty chest infection, recurrent fevers.

"Have you travelled anywhere recently, Cassie?"

She looks at me a bit askance.

"No."

"Anyone else unwell?"

"Well, apart from a room full of five-year-olds, no."

"Okay. Well, we will send some more tests off, keep you on the antibiotics and see you again tomorrow. It looks like a chest infection, but we should do a quick scan of the heart as well."

Cassie's sister's ears prick up at this.

"An echo? When will that happen? Middle of next week or something?"

"I can do a quick one this afternoon?"

Both Cassie and her sister seem a bit more pleased with that.

I wander off to find the echo machine and think a bit more about Cassie. She's in a high-risk group and has a raised heart marker and low markers of white cells – just like the patients at the other hospitals – although her X-ray wasn't very similar at all. Should we test her for coronavirus? I ask myself and decide yes. On the way back with the machine, I ask the nurses to collect a viral swab for the usual viruses, and another one for coronavirus. They aren't sure how to do a swab for coronavirus. I suppose no one here has done it, and I don't know if there's a special bottle. I call microbiology. There's no answer. Then I try virology, and after 12 rings, I get through to a registrar.

"Yes?"

"I was just wondering if we could test a patient up on the heart ward for coronavirus?"

"Any travel?"

"No, but…"

"Any coronavirus contacts?"

"No, but…"

"She doesn't meet the criteria. It'll get refused. Thanks."

I'm left listening to a dial tone. Message received. To be fair, they must be unbelievably busy.

I do the heart scan and it's all reassuringly normal. As I'm finishing the exam, my pager goes off. I give them both a quick explanation of the findings and go off to call back the number. It's intensive care, demanding to know where I've been all day. They need me downstairs now. Knowing better than to ask, I head downstairs, on a hunch wheeling the echo machine with me in the lift and then down the half-dozen floors to this hospital's intensive care department.

One of the biggest intensive cares I've seen in my career, there are over 30 beds down here, and I quickly get lost trying to find the doctors' office. I'm rescued by the ICU matron, and I wheel my machine inside to find the intensive care consultant, Dr Andrews, and a familiar face standing next to him. Sally and I were juniors together, and years ago worked together in the acute medical unit. On slightly different training paths, Sally became an anaesthetist, covering operations and intensive care units, and I went to do hospital medicine and hearts. We lost touch, but bumping into a friend, especially in those lonely safari weekends, is always appreciated.

"Dom!"

"Hello Sally!"

"What are you doing down here?"

"Cardiology. You?" It's a stupid question, given that she's wearing scrubs and standing next to the ICU consultant. She just gestures to herself.

"Sorry, stupid question. You guys have some patients for me?"

Dr Andrews pipes up. In his late fifties, he's short and slim, with a neat cut of white hair atop a kindly face. He's wearing a bright purple bow-tie and brace combo. He looks genuinely happy to see me, which makes a nice change.

"Yes, please. We've got this chap, bacterial pneumonia, diabetes, not in great shape. He was doing well, but then seemed to fall in a heap again. Tube back in, all the works. We asked them to do a heart scan – apparently his heart is a bit puffed. Let us know what you think?"

As referrals go, this is definitely one of the more colourful.

"Of course," I say.

"Splendid! Sally will catch you up."

Dr Andrews strides out purposefully, taking another call from A&E on his mobile. It certainly feels like all systems go here. The unit is already full, but there are no coronavirus cases as yet. Just the usual post-surgical operations, knife and gun wounds and infections. Intensive care departments are usually close to full at the best of times. And it hasn't exactly been the best of times for many years. Sally and I start chatting about her patient. I look at the echo pictures and the blood test results. I recommend a few extra medicines and suggest we do some investigations if he gets off the ventilator. The patient does have a slightly odd history, though.

"His bloods are slightly strange – another infection maybe? It's quite a long time for bacterial pneumonia," I say.

Sally shrugs and jots down the plan. Then she gets a bleep and has to scoot down to A&E to join her boss, as there's another patient to try and bring back up to intensive care.

The hospital feels charged, more so than the last. A controlled manic energy seems to tinge every conversation. Everyone is expecting the wave to hit at any minute. It doesn't take long.

*   *   *

The next morning, I do the hospitals in reverse order, starting where I finished the day before. I'm doing my rounds back on the heart ward when I get a call from Sally. She sounds a little upset.

"Did you see that chap in our ICU? With the poor heart?" she asks me.

I've seen more than a few in the hours between. All had poor hearts.

"The chap we spoke about? Pneumonia got worse again?" I reply.

"Yes. Did you go into his room?"

"Nope. I just documented it and added him to the list to see when he comes out of ICU."

"Oh, okay."

I put two and two together – yesterday was the day we were expecting the routine COVID-19 tests of ICU patients to come back.

"Did he come back with coronavirus?" I ask.

"Yes… I have to go home now. Self-isolate for two weeks."

"Are you okay, Sally?"

"Yeah, fine. Just, well, I intubated him quite a few times. Was definitely exposed. We had no idea."

I try to reassure her.

"It's fine, Sally, you're young, and healthy, and a woman! Best risk group ever."

"I guess," she says.

"And two weeks at home sounds nice."

"Not really," she answers.

"No, I guess not. Let me know if you need anything," I tell her.

"Thanks, Dom." She rings off.

It's not too long after when two rather harassed-looking men arrive on the ward, one a senior doctor I haven't met before, the other a senior manager. They spot me loitering in the corridor between patient rooms.

"Are you the cardiology registrar?" The senior doctor is a ruddy-faced man with a shock of wild grey hair. He's slightly breathless. I get the feeling this is the last stop on what has been a whistle-stop tour of the hospital.

"Yes, I'm Dom."

"Great – we need to find these contacts of the case down-stairs," he says, with urgency, before adding: "COVID-19."

He passes me the list. Both Cassie's and Krish's names are on there.

"Well, I wanted to test Cassie anyway," I told them.

"Oh, why's that?" the doctor asks.

I tell them the story – the two share a look.

"Okay, let's get it done ASAP. Are they both in side rooms?"

I nod.

"Great."

Both swoop off, leaving me very worried about my patients. The nurses ask if someone needs to explain to them before we test. I agree to do it. Krish just shrugs, but Cassie breaks down in tears, desperately worried. I try to reassure her that it's just precautionary. I hope to God it is.

Several of the nurses are now really upset by the possibility of COVID-19 on their ward. Not for the first time I realize that many staff are actually in the high-risk group themselves, overweight, and over 60. I wonder if we shouldn't start shifting everyone over 50 to non-frontline work. A couple of the nurses are talking about having to come into work at the last minute today to cover for three nurses who got sent home to self-isolate for two weeks due to possible contact with the confirmed COVID-19 patient. I wonder how, as the cases keep coming in, that can possibly remain sustainable?

I do the rest of the ward round changing the decisions I made the day before – anyone that can go home gets discharged. We transfer all the scans we can to the outpatients' department; we also make arrangements for follow-up blood tests and ambulatory care reviews. I'm far stricter with any "keep them in just in case" decisions, making sure there's a very stringent benefit to any patient being in the hospital for a minute longer than they need to be. The ward sister and I fight about a patient who hasn't been discharged because they have diarrhoea, but have otherwise completely recovered from the stent inserted in a heart artery 10 days prior. Like all fights with the senior nurses, I do not win. Having managed to discharge half the patients on my list, I feel this isn't a hill I need to die on right now, and there's plenty more to do. Even over the course of the day, the energy in the hospital is building. Something is coming, we all feel it. We can't make out the exact shape of it yet, but it's coming fast. *Too fast.*

• • •

The fever pitch felt in hospitals is starting to seep out into the wider world. On the way home my news feeds are full of videos of fights in supermarkets, which, for reasons still unclear to me, are mostly over toilet paper. I text Dilsan: "Corona cases at the hospital." She pings me back immediately. Like all of us she is glued to her phone most evenings. I make a mental note to get back to trying to cut down social media time.

"Shall we panic buy?" she texts back.

Shockingly, it's a completely legitimate question in the circumstances – it's hard to get to the shops, we have two young children, we don't want to be negligent parents. It's the first of so many surreal moments, contemplating the unthinkable.

"No," I reply, "food transport shouldn't stop, even in a lockdown. It hasn't anywhere else." I really hope I'm not wrong about this.

I swing into the local Tesco on the way home – it's around 8.30 p.m. and the shelves in key areas are almost entirely empty.

A single, misshapen kiwi lurks sadly in an otherwise bare section. There's no toilet paper, the milk is down to specialty coconut milk only and the fresh and ready meals sections are empty, as is the frozen section. The only cans left on the shelf are cannellini beans, and I can't find any sort of pasta anywhere. Thankfully, they have one packet of nappies and some of the baby's formula left, and we have food for a few days at home, at least.

Later, I see all those heartbreaking testimonials of vulnerable elderly shoppers and a picture of an old chap holding a shopping list that simply reads "eggs" next to a cleaned-out shelf, looking utterly bewildered. It's the first time the social contract seems to bend – we're experiencing an event so major that even the absolute basics of normal life are being stretched. It's unnerving. I'm going to be working fairly solidly for the next week, and I'm wondering how we are going to get to the shops in time if it's going to be like this every day.

When I get home, the news is streaming quietly in the background – it's become a nightly obsession now. Italy is announcing a national lockdown, and Germany and France are reportedly doing the same. It's becoming clear the response here is diverging day by day from what other countries are doing, and yet our numbers are similar and at least two patients have already died. The Prime Minister is announcing that he expects "significant" outbreaks.

Dilsan demands I strip at the door and get straight in the shower, and all my clothes go straight in the wash. It seems an utterly bizarre and chilly ritual to maintain after every shift, but I can't argue against it. I have colleagues who are already considering moving out of the home they share with their vulnerable relatives entirely, finding rented accommodation or even hotels. After I shower and eat, we start talking about this, too.

Now that the numbers of COVID patients are rapidly increasing in our hospitals, how do we protect our families? It's a conversation that lurches between the clinical and the irrational; on the one hand, the risk to anyone in our house is very low, but on the other, we don't know in the long term what happens to children. Is it easy to avoid bringing it home? Can I shower at work? Should I move out? The weekend ward rounds, the panic buying, the lockdowns on the news, it all gets too much.

"Shall we just run away?" Dilsan asks, more serious than I realize.

I laugh. "Where would we run to?"

"The country? Your parents?"

"You want to stay at my mum and dad's for the whole pandemic?"

"Well, no." Dilsan gets angrier. "I'm serious, what if you get sick?"

"I'll be fine – I'm low-risk."

"Are you? You're half-Asian, male and, let's face it, could be in better shape."

"I'm 32."

"And a healthcare worker, seeing COVID patients."

"And who would look after the patients in the hospital?"

"Is that more important than our family?"

For a fleeting moment I consider her point. But then an easier way to explain it comes to mind.

"So who would look after my dad, or Ehsan, if they got sick?"

"Well, obviously not you."

"Yes, so some other doctor or nurse would have to. That prioritized their patients over their own family."

Dilsan looks at me balefully. She shrugs.

"So I would look after their family, and they would look after mine. That's the whole point."

We both take a breath.

"I'm just really scared," Dilsan says.

"I am too," I reply.

"I miss Nesli," she adds.

We haven't seen those guys in a few weeks now, and I suddenly get a sinking feeling that we probably won't see them again for a long time. More pressingly, they both currently work in schools, and no one seems to have a clear idea about how infectious children can potentially be. I text Ehsan to remind him to wear his mask and try to avoid the tube.

"Is there any chance you can work from home?" I ask him.

"I can ask the boss, but I doubt it. Schools are still open. What do you think of this?"

He pings me a conversation with some of his friends who are GPs. They're talking about seeing patients with suspected coronavirus in the community with no travel history and being unable to test them – the same situation I'm dealing with in hospital.

"It's the same all over – it's in the community now," I tell him.

"Let me speak to the Head," Ehsan says.

It's hard to convey how worried I am about Ehsan without sounding either hysterical or patriarchal. I'm not sure I really manage it. Solid organ* transplant patients, like Ehsan, appear

---

* Term referring to whole-organ transplants (liver, lung, kidneys, heart, rarely gut) as opposed to an infusion of cells, e.g. stem cell transplant

to be the highest risk group for COVID-19, although there isn't a lot of information about liver transplants. I hope he makes progress with the Head.

In the meantime, Beck has a gig the following day. I have tried to support her career as much as possible and have always been there in the front row of any performance for the last few years. With kids and work it has got trickier, but it's ever-increasingly worth it when I finally can get there; Beck has an incredible talent, and every time I see her perform live she just gets better and better. Her voice is liquid gold, and, knowing so much of the details of her life, her music is so personal to me. Work and kids aside, I'm now really worried about gatherings. Treading lightly given how unwell she was previously, I check in over the phone. She's still having sinusitis-like symptoms, and feeling very under the weather, but no fever or cough. I ask her to think about cancelling, both for her health and that of the audience. She doesn't listen, though, and we chat about other things. Her stage time has been pushed back to 10.30 p.m., so I tell her I'll struggle to make that with an early shift in the morning. Beck doesn't mind – she just wants to get this gig done and then to have some time to recuperate. I invite her to come and live with us again, but she declines. It seems like we are back on our normal good terms, though, and cancelling the family visit last week has been forgotten about.

* * *

I find it hard to sleep that night. I think Dilsan and I both do. I run through a plan to protect Nesli and Ehsan, to look after my Dad and to try and prepare things at work. The thoughts rattle around in my head like ice in a cocktail shaker. Zach wakes up at 3 a.m., and I get up and settle him, before diverting myself downstairs to make a cup of peppermint tea. I try and write a little, look up houseboat prices, wondering if that's where we should be moving to, and search for the latest infection numbers from Italy, Germany and France again. Outside in the dawn twilight, the first birds chirp quietly. The house is still and quiet. I sit curled up on the couch in a pool of soft lamplight, the laptop open. This should be a peaceful time, but I'm restless, agitated. I come across a news article from the UK about shortages of personal protective equipment being reported at some hospitals. The crisis hasn't even begun, and already the threads of the system are fraying, unattended.

At that point it was still considered sensationalist to discuss COVID in terms of a war – scaremongering, in fact. The irony is that we'd spent previous years using the language of the last world war in our politics with abandon, and yet faced with a comparable crisis, we suddenly found restraint. Thinking of my conversations with Dilsan and Ehsan, bunkered in our houses against an unseen enemy, there were parallels with the Blitz. We could see the distant front, in continental Europe, unfolding live on our screens. The accounts from Italy were terrifying – overwhelmed hospitals with broken staff, the complete abandonment of normal practices just to survive, and placing 16 million people under quarantine.

It occurred to me then that the country needed to fundamentally rethink its approach to COVID-19. Less a storm in a teacup, or even a storm that will blow over, but a prolonged and protracted conflict. The more I looked at our own case figures, doubling roughly every three days, the more it seemed our trajectory became terminal. Around 43,000 men and women lost their lives in the Blitz. COVID-19 could be worse. That day (8 March), the total of confirmed cases reached 278, and by that maths, there would be over 400 by mid-week, and over 1,000 cases by the following week. Without drastic intervention, the pandemic would continue at the same pace for weeks and weeks. And the question no one was asking was how will we provide the same urgent and emergency care when we are overwhelmed by COVID-19 in each hospital? The simple answer: we won't. We can cancel elective work and waiting list operations, but those patients don't disappear, and neither do their health needs. COVID-19 deaths will be fastidiously documented, but what about these indirect mortalities from delays and diverted care because of the pandemic? The knock-on effect will be devastating and incalculable.

I decide, sat there with my tea, that this will be akin to the Blitz, and that we need to start thinking of it like that. A marathon, not a sprint. There's no point panic buying, you are only impoverishing others, and this will last months, if not years. The more I think about it, the more the slogans my gran used to tell me about World War Two seem so apt in this situation: "Loose lips sink ships" – misinformation and conspiracy theories will sink us as surely now as they did then. We need to listen and follow advice. "Dig for victory" – we need to dig deep and be resourceful and self-reliant, to go the extra mile and keep going. "Keep calm and carry on" – we have to face this with clear eyes and open hearts. We can survive this, but only together.

It occurs to me in that quiet moment that I need to make a will, we both do. The sun breaks over the garden fence and spreads yellow-orange fingers into the living room. Max, our cat, saunters in and springs up next to me, massaging his claws into the blanket and purring loudly as I scratch the nape of his neck through his thick blue-grey fur. Pensively I sit there, making plans, scrapping them, and starting again.

CHAPTER 5

Escalation

After the weekend, I've got a rare half-day off; I've just got a clinic to cover in the morning. A friend of a friend just posted on one of our WhatsApp groups that he flew in from Lombardy last night, without so much as a check or even a question from the officials at Heathrow, and got straight onto the tube. As I sit in the carriage, my hands are firmly lodged in my jacket and my mask sits snugly on my face. I still feel uncomfortable. Having hardly slept, I'm starting to feel very tired. I crawl into the coffee shop by the tube station and cling to the cup as if it's holding me up. I was only here 16 hours ago, but things are moving so fast now that the hospital feels materially different again: quieter, thinner crowds in the atrium, a subdued buzz of those doing what they can, quietly worried.

The boss in the clinic today is Dr Rich Porter. A young consultant and a high-flying academic, he is already well on his way to professorship. We've worked together a few times before, and besides being razor-sharp, Rich is also one of the nicest cardiology consultants I've met. He is someone that I've been chatting to about a potential research job (for my PhD), and I drop in to catch up before the clinic starts.

"Morning," I say.

Rich glances up from his laptop.

"Oh, hi, Dom." He gives me a look. "You okay?"

"Not really sleeping. How are you?"

"Did you see this?" he replies, diverted by an online news article. "Retired docs recalled to frontline."

"It's inevitable, I guess. Be interested to see how they convince the most at-risk groups to come back to the most high-risk areas, though."

"If they're pulling them in, then they'll be pulling doctors out of research, too."

Thinking of my colleagues who have just left for PhDs, I realize that they will all be back shortly too. I try to wrangle the conversation back to something more positive. "Any news on the research job?"

I've been waiting to hear back about this PhD for months already.

"I'll chase them up – it's looking good!" he tells me.

I just give a wry little laugh. The world of academia is so alien to me, I'm still learning the rules. So far, I've gathered that "right away" means "maybe in the next few months", "I'm interested" means "Do you have any money?" and "Let's see what we can do" means "Go and find some money". You'd imagine a world driven by esoteric pursuits of lofty ideals and science, but the system is driven by results and by publications, and results need money, in the form of grants and funding. It can be quite dog-eat-dog – academics who don't deliver routinely lose their jobs. I've learnt to be patient. We get the clinic started.

Judging the mood, in the newspapers and outside, I'm expecting a few patients to simply not turn up – what we call Did Not Attend (DNA). Given the risk of coming into hospital on tubes and buses, crossing busy streets and sitting in waiting rooms, at some point we will need to stop doing these clinics entirely. Some hospitals have already started telephoning their patients at home instead, an idea that caused uproar among traditional medics only a few months ago when it was mooted as a way to improve the service and make it more efficient. The lack of physical examination, of non-verbal communication, of rapport – the list of problems with it had been endless. But then COVID-19 hit, and what was formerly a radical and unpopular idea became, overnight, the only logical solution, even a popular one. Now I'm being told that patients really like telephone consultations in general – it's far more convenient and saves valuable time for all parties. We've known for hundreds of years that most of the diagnosis is made in simply talking to people, as much as 80 per cent; the physical examination is only 10 per cent and tests and investigations even less. I wonder if this change will endure in the long term, when the crisis is over.

I have a look down the list for today – there aren't that many patients, and at least one has requested a telephone appointment. I see a patient pop on the system to tell me they have (physically) arrived. I pull up her notes.

Janet is in her mid-sixties and has retired, having run a laundromat empire for most of her life. A year ago, she was taking the bins out when she felt some chest tightness and soon collapsed. In A&E, the assessing doctor found a murmur and sent her to see us shortly afterwards. We ordered a heart scan, which showed a tightening of the main valve pumping blood out of the heart, the aortic valve. The normal aortic valve is a thing of beauty, comprizing three cusps, or "leaflets", each a delicate curve of sinewy tissue, which together form a perfect replica of the Mercedes-Benz logo. Each beat of the heart pushes a column of blood past the valve, and the cusps flip open and then snap back again, meeting perfectly in the middle. Janet's aortic valve did not feature those pristine loops of tissue; over time, it had become gnarled and calcified, stiffened and unable to open fully, increasing the pressure required to open it. Eventually, this led to her chest pain and collapse.

There are a few letters on the system about Janet. One of my colleagues who saw her last year sent her to see a cardio-thoracic surgeon to consider a heart operation. But there are no further letters on the system about it, and she is back here again. Somewhere this has gone awry. I check her appointments, though, and see that she is scheduled to see one of the surgeons next week.

I call her in. "Mrs Fife."

Janet is dressed in a woollen cardigan and stands up cheerily. She gives me a little wave and picks up about four bags she has collected around her, before shuffling into my clinic room. She offers her hand to shake, and we have a slightly awkward impasse where I don't take it.

"Coronavirus, you know," I say, offering her my elbow, but she doesn't understand. I should probably work on this, I think to myself. Janet is unfazed and flumps down in the clinic chair.

"How are you?" is her first question.

I laugh. I can't help it, it's such a strange role reversal. It breaks the ice. The whole formal consultation takes less than five minutes. I check her heart scan, which shows that her heart valve is severely thickened. She doesn't have any new symptoms, and still wants to have surgery. Nothing has changed. I make a conscious choice to not examine her – I can't justify additional contact when it won't change anything that we do. Like so many of the patients I see that day, Janet needn't have come all the way into the hospital to see me. This is the perfect example of a situation in which a telephone appointment would have easily sufficed.

There's no one else to see so we just chat a little. We fill the time talking about nothing in particular, my kids, her grand-kids, east London, Camden Market. A lifelong Londoner, Janet has some great stories. We wrap up, laugh about the lack of a handshake a second time, and I usher her out from a safe distance. As Janet makes her way out, a man in his early twen-ties is hovering sheepishly outside and leaps aside to let her pass. Clutching a notebook, and with a fearfully expectant manner, he catches my eye.

"HelloI'mAMedicalStudentCanIJoinYourClinic?" he blurts out, without pauses.

I remember those days well, bouncing from foot to foot, waiting for the boss to open the door. Trying to catch up and learn from a new stranger teaching you nearly every day, while desperately trying not to get in the way.

"Sure, medical student, do you have a name?" I ask, jokingly.

He grins.

"Oki."

"Great, first year clinical?"

"Yes."

"Cool, take a seat."

I go through Janet's case quickly, highlighting the various teaching points. Thinking of the pandemic, I ask Oki about what the medical school is doing to prepare them.

"Prepare us for what?" he asks.

"For coronavirus? Is there a plan for you guys? Maybe for the final-year students?"

"How do you mean, plan? I'm going on holiday in three weeks."

"Um. I don't think you are," I say, suspecting that everyone's going to be drafted in to help. "What has the medical school told you?"

"Nothing, really. No changes."

I find this all quite worrying and I wonder what's happening behind the scenes. Not wanting to convey my anxiety to Oki, we move back to talking about Janet, and how we probably aren't doing enough to determine which patients really need to be physically seen. We get the next patient in. The rest of the clinic is depressingly similar – so many of these patients needn't have travelled across London to see us today. Like the 80-year-old retired gardener who had triple-bypass surgery 20 years ago, who, for some inexplicable reason, we have been seeing every year to check up on. He remains completely asymptomatic, as he has for years. I offer to discharge him, but he would rather come back annually – I can't seem to talk him out of this but write down "for possible telephone appt next time", wondering if we'll still be doing it in a year's time.

There's also a young secretary who has a sister with a bicuspid aortic valve (meaning she has only two valve leaflets instead of the usual three) – it's a congenital defect that can affect members of the same family. These valves are prone to becoming stiff and damaged much faster, so, like Janet, her sister ended up needing a valve replacement, but, unlike Janet, her sister was only 40 at the time. The young secretary's GP has referred her for screening for the same heart condition. I examine her carefully but can't hear anything wrong. I ask Oki to examine her as well, and we're careful to wash our hands first. I ask him if he heard anything, wondering if he'll confabulate a heart murmur. He does admirably, declaring, "I couldn't hear any murmurs." I am pleased, but the patient will need an echocardiogram anyway.

The end of the clinic comes quicker than normal, as we've had several non-attendees, and the one telephone patient ironically didn't pick up. Rich tells me he left a voicemail but doesn't really know what the etiquette is with telephone appointments. We normally won't see patients that come in over 30 minutes late – there simply isn't room in the schedule. Do we call them back later? Neither of us knows. Everything is changing on the fly and we are trying to keep up. It feels like COVID is shaking the whole system and all the outdated or unnecessary practices are crumbling off. Perhaps face-to-face clinic appointments will be one of those. Oki makes his excuses and disappears to find his next teacher.

Rich is with the last patient as I'm finishing. I pop my head in to check we are finished, and he waves me off – he's actually trying to phone back the telephone patient again. I check in on a few of the patients from the weekend remotely – the guidelines for testing COVID-19 patients changed that morning, and now we can finally test patients who haven't travelled, nearly 11 days after the first community case was recorded. Two of the suspected patients from the weekend – Cassie and Krish – have been tested, and thankfully both came back negative. The third case, a young woman with suspicious clinical symptoms, is positive, however, and has been in the hospital for a few days already, although in a side room at least. It's progress, I suppose, but I wonder how many other patients and staff have been unwittingly exposed to coronavirus as a result of this policy.

Outside, the weather is turning; it's milder but still bracing, and a gust whips my jacket as I trudge toward the tube. I'm dreading the afternoon, for a specific and rather selfish reason: I have to shave my beard.

● ● ●

We had an email round last week, inviting all the on-call teams to get "fit tested" for the masks that we will need to wear when in contact with COVID-19 patients. This strikes me as strange, as it's the first time in eight years I've ever heard of this in hospitals, and I wonder if we are to be issued with specific military-style masks, imagining a full-face gas mask with bulging canisters and leather straps – a terrifying sight for the patients. I find out that actually it's the law to undergo "fit testing" for all filtering facepiece masks – a way of making sure that the specific shape and size of mask fits your face exactly with a tight enough seal to not allow air in or out. It's something I haven't really considered for the filtering facepiece mask I've been wearing to and from work every day.

The test is very strict. No food or drink for one hour before (although I can't see why), and men need to be completely clean-shaven. There isn't any specific instruction for what "clean-shaven" means. Fresh from the barber? A five o'clock shadow? A few days' growth? I've worn a beard for nearly the whole 13 years I've been with Dilsan, and on the few occasions I've had to shave it entirely, she tells me I look like an alien and won't look directly at me until it grows back. The kids have never seen me without a beard. Due for a fit test in the morning, I have to go and buy a razor again, something I haven't done for a decade. I buy the exact same one I had when I was 13, a Gillette Mach something.

When I tell Dilsan the sad news about my facial hair, she is devastated.

"Will you have to keep it like that?" she asks.

"Yes, I guess."

"Well, you will probably need to move out then."

She's only half-joking.

I spend some time saying a long goodbye to what my daughter refers to as "my whiskers". I shave my beard into some prospector-style sideburns, have a go at a Tony Stark moustache and goatee combo, mess it up, and then shave the whole thing clean, cutting myself repeatedly through lack of practice. I leave my sideburns too long and feel I've lost about 15 years in age and several decades in fashion. I tiptoe down with trepidation to show Dilsan. Her face is genuinely upset.

"I hate it."

I'm expecting this, but it's just another strangeness in what has been a torrent of the surreal. It's also the first material thing that has changed at home. When the outside world was sliding so quickly into crisis, our house remained an untouched oasis. It was easy to pretend, even for a little while, that everything was normal. But my newly shorn cheeks are a constant and drastic reminder of how everything is changing. The reviews from the kids the next morning are equally crushing. Ayla is very blunt about it; when she sees me, she simply says:

"You are not my daddy anymore."

Oof.

Zach is cutting. His vocabulary is still pretty limited to "Da", but he makes his feelings known just the same. When he sees me come into the kitchen, he looks directly at me, and then very deliberately turns his head to look away when I come to give him a kiss.

Dilsan laughs, and so do I. It's cute, but I can't help feeling a little upset by it all as well. My Twitter feed that morning on the way to work is filled with similarly laughably pathetic stories from male colleagues up and down the country. It's a strange sort of solidarity across the network, an acknowledgement that we are all getting ready for something. I read that apparently a moustache is considered acceptable facial hair to pass the fit test, so I make a mental note for the next time, although I'm not sure that will go down any better at home.

The next morning, my first stop is the fit-test clinic, but when I get there, there's already a queue snaking around the corridor. I tried to get an appointment last week, and heard by word of mouth it was in one part of the building only to find nothing there, and then chased it up again in the new location only to be turned away for not having an appointment. This time I have a pre-arranged time: 9.15 a.m. I'm five minutes early. I knock on the door, and a harassed-looking nurse pops her head round. "Do you have an appointment?" she snaps. "Um, yes, 9.15 a.m." She checks her notepad.

"Ah yes. We are overbooked. Can you come back this afternoon?" she asks.

I tsk. I'm actually off today and had planned to go home to write grant proposals for my research. The fit test was the sole reason I came in, but I'm on-call the coming weekend and will have little opportunity in the week to return. Imagining some special mask will be delivered to me at the end of this process, I trudge off with an appointment rebooked for 1.15 p.m.

There's a meeting at midday to discuss COVID preparations with the other registrars, several of whom dial in to the meeting on an app I've never heard of called Zoom. I shuffle in and sit in the corner. The senior consultant I don't know well, but he is in charge of a few of the services for the entire trust. He summarizes the situation: that the official "expectation" will be a significant patient load as we are already seeing many cases in the other hospitals. So far, we as a group don't have any specific changes to action, but we're told that routine activity will likely reduce in the next few weeks as cases increase and that telephone clinics will very shortly become the norm. He asks if we have any questions. I ask about moving between hospitals, and when that will stop. There are no immediate plans. We also discuss the need to cross-train staff, especially intensive care staff. There's some nodding, but I can see it's not really landing with some of the others. There are a few scrambled questions from the registrars via Zoom, which are hard to make out, and then the meeting is done. Everything feels like it's moving so slowly. Too slowly.

I nip back downstairs to my fit-test appointment, knock on the door again, and am told they are running late and to return at 2.45 p.m. A group of six or seven doctors, nurses, radiographers and physiotherapists are already clustered around the door.

"When was your appointment?" I ask a physio I know from the wards.

"12 p.m." He shrugs.

I wander off slightly aimlessly, before gravitating toward the library. I manage to write about three words of a grant proposal before it's time to go back upstairs again. The prospect of research seems so unlikely to me now that the song and dance of writing a proposal seems farcical anyway. Meanwhile, Dilsan is texting me wondering what's happened to my "quick morning trip to work".

By mid-afternoon, it's been about 20 hours since my last shave and my jaw is sporting half a five o'clock shadow.

I knock on the door, for the fourth time.

"Yes?"

"I have an appointment at 2.45 p.m., I think?"

"Name?"

"Dominic. Pimenta."

"Nope. Can you call the number?"

"Sorry, it was supposed to be at 1.15 and you pushed it back?"

"Oh. Yes. Okay. Come in."

The room is set up with a computer wrapped in a suitcase-like shell, with a tube snaking to a hard mask I haven't seen before.

There's another nurse in there.

"Hold up, you need to have shaved."

"I did. Last night."

"There's a diagram on the door, did you not read it?"

"I did. It said no beards. I don't have a beard."

"We can't test you like that."

"So how recently do I need to have shaved?"

"Did you not see the diagram?"

"Yes, it didn't help. Is it six hours? Twelve hours?"

"It was in the email."

"I was here this morning and no one mentioned it."

"It was in the email."

"I didn't get any email."

"The emails were disseminated by the department heads."

"I didn't get an email."

"The emails were dis—"

"Can you send me the email then? So I can see the instructions clearly?"

"The emails were disseminated by the department heads."

I feel like I've walked into a real-life re-enactment of *Catch-22*. I look pleadingly around at the other people in the room.

"Does anyone have this email? Can I see it? Can you send it to me?" I ask, despairingly.

"You will need to email your department head, to get the email."

I take a deep breath. I give up trying to understand the rules around shaving and make another appointment for tomorrow, between clinics. Outside, I find one of the junior nurses from the ward, Kelvin.

"Hey, Kelvin – do you have this email about fit-testing?"

"Oh, yeah, sure." He pulls out his phone and pings me a copy.

I pick it up on my phone and look through it. It's the same diagram as on the door outside, with no extra information.

This process has been so dehumanizing, a product of trying to get as many people through the testing as quickly as possible, in the limited time we now have. I head home, deflated. I reflect that if we are going to be asked to risk our lives, the least we can expect is to be treated like people. We are trying to operate in a critical emergency using the same infrastructure we had before. We need to do a whole bunch of things, as quickly as possible, things we have never really had to do before: have a way to contact all staff simultaneously, collect into staff groups for quick messaging, have multiple layers of contact as well as direct ones, be able to rapidly feed back from the ground to the decision-making body, cross-train staff, consider cohorting staff in high-risk groups and organize patients into "negative", "suspected" and "positive" areas. Italian hospitals in the north are now in full meltdown, and they started lockdown measures, like closing schools, when they had only 322 cases. I check our case number for today. It's 321. So, we're roughly 10–14 days behind Italy and we are now passing the milestones left ahead of us and ignoring each one as we plough forwards. On the tube home, I manically scribble down every thought I have about all this.

Hunched on the platform waiting for a connecting train, my face is strangely cold. Each passing minute begins to feel like another missed opportunity to take positive action, and as cases are now doubling every two days, our response needs to reflect that. We are ignoring all the warning signs, not just from Italy, but also from the World Health Organization. It seems more and more as if the government is pursuing the "herd immunity" plan, no matter the wave of patients that would break on our hospitals and care homes – the wave that would break on top of me and my colleagues.

* * *

Digesting the thoughts from the previous day, on the next morning, Wednesday 11 March, I tweeted: "If #coronavirusuk continues similarly to Italy we have perhaps 10 days before we reach meltdown in hospitals, medical students have had no briefing, retired docs have no plans to return, there has been no cross-training of staff, we only started testing community pts yesterday."

The tweet resonates instantly, and takes me by surprise. This also happens on the same morning as the news reports that a government minister has now tested positive for COVID-19. Social media is alight with the threat COVID poses, and yet everywhere else seems nearly blasé in comparison. Doctors, too, like some in Dilsan's social media groups, plan to go skiing or are thinking about the rota in a month's time. It's not just woolly thinking, it's something else. A wilful need to not look objectively at the numbers.

The stories from Italy terrify me: pathologists who haven't looked after an unwell patient in decades are being dumped on the frontline running non-invasive ventilation, because the health system has simply run out of any other clinical staff. Some reports indicate that doctors are forced to choose who to save, with those over 65 not even being assessed by intensive care departments. Every diagnosis is the same: bilateral pneumonia, COVID-19.

Given these accounts, I can't understand the inaction on our end. I watched Professor Chris Whitty's testimony at the Health and Social Care Select Committee on 6th March again, to which Boris Johnson later responded that it was important not to "fire your shots too early" in escalating measures to tackle the illness. I get the logic of "going too early" when it comes to lockdown measures and interventions in terms of the potential business and economic impact, but it feels as though we're going to have to decide what's more important: livelihoods or lives. They need to throw resources at this now, not wait until we have to let patient after patient just drop dead in front of us.

I decide then that I should really start to keep a diary. I'm really bad at emotions. I get stomach bleeds and muscle twitches instead of feeling stressed. And then sometimes I'll just snap, maybe once every few years, and break down for a day. Then I pick myself up and I'm back to it. Somehow, I don't think that'll cut it this time. I feel like I'm losing my mind, and yet when I go to work, it's some of my colleagues that don't seem willing to accept reality, to see what is happening in front of our eyes. I feel like Cassandra, from Greek mythology, who was cursed to never have her warnings heeded and to always feel like no one was listening. I lost faith long ago in the government and know that our Senior NHS administrators, many of whom are political animals and not clinical ones, are fallible like anyone else.

The mortality rate among 30- to 40-year-olds is 0.2 per cent. That's based on a flawed case definition that does not include patients with mild symptoms, meaning the chance of getting really sick if you get infected is hopefully even lower than that. But that's still 1 in 500 30-year-olds who will die from this. If 50 million are infected, how many my age will die? Will *I* die? Maybe.

I've been reading my Bible fairly regularly by this point. I don't read it as gospel, ironically. I'm looking for something in it I can't quite explain yet, a shape of a life I think we should all lead, of the kind of person I want to be. Respectful, kind, brave, believing. Contrary to the prevailing politics of today, Jesus turns out to be a tub-thumping socialist. He turfed the money-lenders out of the Church, hated the hypocrites in the Temple and wanted everyone to stop talking about their faith and actually practise it by going and praying in private. Maybe when he said "I am the way" he meant "Live like I did", first and foremost. When I pick up my leather Gideon Bible now, it's like a balm compared to the angry blue light of my smart-phone. I think more and more that I'll be coming back to my Bible in the coming months.

· · ·

When I get home Dilsan is ashen-faced and close to tears, trying to hold it together as she speaks down the phone.

"Don't worry, Nesli, it'll be okay," she says, looking up as I come in the door. "Dom's home – I'll call you back."

"What's wrong?" I ask.

"Ehsan is sick," she says.

The words are like a slap in the face, knocking out the frustrations of the day.

"He has a runny nose, sore eyes, and feels tired."

"Temperature?"

"The highest Nesli could get was 37.7°C."

"Any cough? Or breathing issues?"

Dilsan shakes her head.

The isolation guidelines are limited to fever and cough, but I don't really know what COVID-19 might look like in someone on immunosuppressant drugs, and certainly 37.7°C could be considered a low-grade fever, especially on those same drugs.

"Ehsan should call the helpline, but needs to self-isolate," I say.

To be honest, he should probably be self-isolating anyway at this point, but there's no official guidance and the government doesn't look anywhere close to closing schools, where both Nes and Ehsan work.

Dilsan looks frightened. I try to reassure her.

"It just sounds like a cold, okay, but make sure he calls the helpline or his GP in the morning, I guess. Tomorrow he can call the liver team and ask them as well."

We get them back on the phone and have a little family conference. Ehsan is feeling better, but it's clear this episode has shaken them both; they've crossed through the looking glass beyond cautious denial. Suddenly they are looking down the barrel of COVID, from the point of view of a family with a highly vulnerable individual, and two young children, working in schools. We chat through the plans.

"They will have to lock down eventually," I say, only 70 per cent sure this is the case. Evidence to date has been to the contrary, but I wonder how long it can go on like this.

"Yeah, but they still might not close the schools."

"You won't be able to go in anyway, Ehsan – you'll need some sort of letter from your liver team, I think."

I have no idea what they are planning for highly vulnerable adults, but it's clear Ehsan needs to avoid leaving the house now as much as possible.

"You have seven days of self-isolation anyway – and then you'll have to see what happens."

"Will they lock down next week, do you think? What if they don't?"

All the once-radical ideas have become options on the table; hiding out in a campervan, Nesli and the boys moving in with us, or even just Nesli, splitting their family up for months, potentially. The conversation ranges from the fearful to the ridiculous; at one point we look up prices on houseboat rentals – an idea I'd been mulling earlier on – and where to sail to. Despite the content, it's actually quite a positive conversation, even if in a slightly forced, overly cheery way. I imagine it's one of tens of thousands of similar conversations that are happening and will happen over the next few weeks around the country, around the world.

"Whatever happens, we will sort it out," says Dilsan. I think her big sisterly role has been beneficial for her own mood. She seems more determined, more purposeful.

"Let's get that letter from your liver team and take it from there," I suggest.

"Let us know how you're feeling, Ehsan, and if you need anything," Dilsan adds into the speakerphone.

"Okay. Love you guys. Night." Ehsan and Nesli ring off.

It's well past midnight.

"What are we going to do?" Dilsan asks again, this time more unsure.

I shrug, imagining that the answer to that question is the same as it would be for any family right now.

"Whatever we can."

. . .

Later in the evening I can't help but think how many vulnerable people like Ehsan are out there, taking unnecessary risks, blissfully unaware of what is coming down the line. I don't want to scare anyone, but equally the national conversation just doesn't match what we are seeing and expecting on the ground. Informed consent is the bedrock of medicine – a patient can only make a legally sound decision about their own health with the right information. I start writing some of these thoughts into another article, a warning to the public and a call to action to the government, to throw everything we have at this, every resource, right now, with no more delay. Training up existing staff, retired doctors (with suitable precautions) and students like Oki, resourcing hospitals with every scrap of PPE and ventilation equipment we can find and providing the public with the means to help contain the epidemic: handwashing areas at transit hubs, supplies at food banks, mass disinfection of public transport. Every second lost feels like it will cost lives.

As I'm writing this, it occurs to me that Dilsan and I haven't finalized our wills. I read it back. It's quite inflammatory, but deliberately so. I send it to a contact at the *Independent* and ask if they will publish it anonymously. I change a few details to mask myself a little more. I want to get the word out with this, but I want to keep my job and not get caught up in the politics that too often dominates large hospital institutions. The *Independent* offers some edits and accepts it straight away. They print it the very next day.

. . .

The next morning I'm in the echo (echocardiogram) department, learning to perform echos (also known as heart ultrasounds, not be confused with ECGs, which are electrocardiograms, and print 2D sheets of the electrical rhythm of the heart). I've got about 500 cases in my logbook and I'm trying to figure out how to finalize the paperwork to get this signed off, which means a lot of hanging around the offices and waiting for the senior technician to have time to look at it. While I'm down there, I start chatting to some of the echocardiographers, the specially trained physiologists who do many of the cardiac jobs in the hospital and don't get nearly enough recognition for them. Their training is very specialist, however, and when it comes to COVID-19, it's as new to them as anybody else. Many are very worried.

Jack is the senior echocardiographer and is sporting a dust mask that his mum bought from the local Halfords. The department has also been issued with surgical masks and full-face shields, although no one is clear if and when they should be used. Doing an echo involves lying the patient on their left-hand side and placing a wand on their chest, needing to get very close beside them to do so. The procedure can last up to 20–25 minutes, so the exposure time is considerable. They have asked us to question every patient on the list before they come in, to find out if they are unwell or have had any unwell contacts. So far, no one has declared themselves a risk and the morning is running very quickly, with lots of waiting time between patients.

Myself and another registrar, Aidan, are working on our logbooks in the main office. Jack is going through the ward requests for echos.

"Dom, do me a favour, mate, can you have a look through these?"

I'm just twiddling my thumbs so happy to help. "Sure, what do you need?"

"Can you vet these for us? Do they all need doing?"

It's not a task I'm keen on – I know all too well the frustration of asking for a scan when I'm in another department and then being interrogated to find out exactly why. Equally, Jack is looking quite anxious, a feeling mirrored on the faces of several of the physiologists down here. Somewhat reluctantly, I pull the stack of paper requests toward me and look through them, working through the electronic system as I do. Just like when I'm in the outpatients' clinic, in the cold light of need, many of these requests actually don't need to be done. Where there is a good reason to perform an echo, often it's only to answer a specific question, so a focused five-minute exam can be done rather than a full 20-minute one, reducing exposure time considerably. The last patient makes me pause.

"Don't do this one," I tell Jack.

"Okay, what shall I write on the form?"

I've got the request and the blood tests up on my screen; the patient, who came in overnight, is a young woman in her mid-thirties with chest pain worse when she breathes in and out. Her inflammatory markers in her blood tests are high and her lymphocytes and platelets are low. I notice her oxygen looks a little low in the notes too. I pull up her chest X-ray – it's subtle, but all points to a pattern we've seen over and over already and will see over and over again. Her last entry in the notes mentions a fever. The echo request had been for suspected pericarditis, an inflammation of the lining of the outside of the heart.

I find the ward phone and ask to speak to the doctor who requested the echo, an SHO named Piotr. Luckily, I've worked with him once or twice before.

"Hello?" Piotr answers.

"Oh, hi, Piotr, this is Dom."

"Oh, hi, Dom."

"Did you guys request an echo for the lady in bed 10?"

"Um…" he begins. There's a rustle of paper on the other end of the phone. "Yes, the pericarditis lady from overnight?"

"I'm just vetting the inpatient echos – could you check with the consultant if this scan is needed to confirm a diagnosis of pericarditis?"

"Oh yeah, probably not." Piotr makes a scribble on the other end. "I'll ask him shortly. Okay, thanks."

"Sorry, Piotr, before you go, did the patient get swabbed for flu, or COVID?"

"There's no travel history, so we didn't do the COVID."

"The guidelines changed three days ago – we should test the community patients who are suspicious, and the bloods and X-ray are suspicious at least."

"Um, okay." Piotr is trying not to be rude, but clearly thinks I'm mad.

"Can you ask the nurses to swab her at least – isn't she in an open bay?"

Open bays are larger areas with four to six beds in them, as opposed to the single side rooms.

"Yeah, sure. Okay, thanks, Dom."

Piotr hangs up. I suspect my request will be way down his list of priorities.

Jack is grateful, but I'm slightly frustrated. I go and grab a coffee.

On my way back one of my bosses calls me. Dr Geffers is in charge of a large clinical area, covering several different hospitals. We are usually on good terms, and have worked together on a few projects in the past. A call out of the blue could mean anything. I go out and find reception and pick up.

"Hi, Phil."

"Dominic," comes the reply. Using my full name is rarely a good start to anything. "I've just been shown one of your tweets." He begins to read it out. "'Hospitals will be in meltdown in 10 days, medical students have had no briefing, there's no cross-training of staff, no plan to bring back retired docs' – now, do you really think that's helpful?"

Phil sounds pretty pissed off, and in normal times this would be a very short, one-way conversation. Slightly perturbed to be called about this, but also very concerned about the wider situation, I push back a little more than I normally would.

"I see your point, Phil – happy to take it down. Is any of it not true, though?"

Phil pauses, and actually seems to think about it before answering: "I've got friends in Lombardy, and yes, it sounds pretty horrendous there, probably about two weeks ahead of us."

"I mean, I don't want to ruffle feathers, but equally we could be doing more here, right?" I say.

Again, this is turning into a strange conversation, as Phil pauses to think on it more.

"Well, bringing back retired docs – good luck to them on that one. What do you mean about cross-training of staff?"

"Maybe some of the medical registrars will need some ventilator training, maybe even go to intensive care? I mentioned it at the briefing."

"Mmm… Yes, I'll speak to Duncan about that." He means Duncan Desmond, one of the lead consultants in intensive care.

"Sorry, Phil, I'm just really worried about this stuff."

"No, it's good. Leave it up, you haven't said anything that isn't in the public eye already and it's all accurate. We could get something more constructive alongside it, though, don't you think?"

"Yes, I suppose – what did you have in mind?"

"Let me think. Might be useful to use your social platform."

"Seriously, anything to help. I'm going crazy wanting to do something."

"Yes, I can see that," Phil says, with less heat and more lightness in his voice now. "Okay, let me get back to you. Cheers, Dom."

He rings off. That was a stranger conversation than I had thought it was going to be.

I cook up a few short tweets about hospital preparedness, some of the general things we are doing, and send it to Phil to have a look. I attach my other rambling pages about various ideas and how we should be doing them. Phil pings back a thumbs up emoji. I take that to mean to send out the tweets and he'll have a look at the rest, but I don't get anything further back from him.

· · ·

When I get back to the echo department, the physiologists have all dispersed to do various scans around the building, and only me and Aidan are left. Aidan is at a similar level to me, about to take a break and go and do his own carefully planned research in Denmark. We get chatting about COVID – by now the subject dominating most conversations in hospitals, it seems.

"Well, I'll be out in Copenhagen in three weeks, so it won't really affect me." Aidan seems super certain about this.

"I think that might be unlikely, mate, if I'm honest. Research will be cancelled, I'd imagine."

"No, they've already spun up the cell lines for me, they're all cooking and ready to go."

"I don't think COVID will care about that. Sorry."

"It won't be that bad, will it, though? I mean, there's only so many beds?"

"We'll get redeployed, or they'll put patients on floors, or get extra beds."

"Nooooo. It'll just blow over, I think."

"Why? Genuinely? Why do you think that?"

"Why wouldn't it?"

"Well, if the case numbers are still doubling every two to three days, and we aren't doing anything to stop that now, then here, look (I show him the document I've been working on): 300 cases yesterday, 600 by Sunday, 1,200 on Tuesday, 2,400 by Friday. In three weeks, we're talking hundreds of thousands. Italy is closed, Aidan!"

Aidan isn't fazed. He's an incredibly smart guy, keen and motivated, but his heart is set on his research and he simply won't listen.

"What part of that do you find reassuring?" I ask.

"I don't, really," he concedes.

"So why don't you think it's going to happen?"

Aidan pauses, genuinely thinking about it. "I suppose a combination of optimism and naivety," he pronounces.

At least he has insight.

It's nearly lunchtime and I have to head upstairs for a fit test, again. I'm already starving, and the appointment time can't come around fast enough. It's a different nurse today, and she doesn't bat an eyelid at my stubble.

"Okay, pop on the mask there."

It's a hard mask I haven't used before, with a tube snaking back to that familiar computer in a box. It looks like a lie detector test in some ways, with a little oscillating display veering between red and green. They get me to do a whole selection of moving and breathing exercises, each time trying to keep the little ticker firmly in the green. It takes about twenty minutes to get through all of it, including a hairy two minutes teetering on the border between the two, when leaning forward. Eventually, I pass.

"So, this is my mask?" I ask, still slightly confused by this.

"Oh, you can take that one with you, but it has a hole in it for the test."

"So, I should try and find this particular one when I need one?"

"Yes, this size."

"Okay, thanks."

Feeling vaguely like I've achieved something but unsure of exactly what, I disappear up to the clinic, taking 10 minutes to grab a sandwich and post the short thread about hospital preparedness that Dr Geffers suggested. What breaks the paralyzing anxiety about the future is physical action toward it, even if the steps are small. Feeling useful, even if in the tiniest way, drives that energy into something else, so it doesn't burn me up. Slightly uplifted, I finish the telephone clinic and head home.

Dilsan texts me to ask me if I'll draft a letter for Ehsan's liver team, with the specific question and wording a highly vulnerable person might need. It's unbelievable that there isn't something in the public domain, especially as London becomes ever increasingly an epidemic centre in itself. I suppose the two questions that need answering are: can you officially confirm that Ehsan is higher risk as a solid organ transplant recipient?; and, is there a sensible length of time to recommend to self-isolate until it's considered safe? Even as I'm drafting this, I imagine receiving the same letter for a heart transplant patient, and wonder how I would handle it. I could phone a specialist, but who could advise on the risk of a new infection in this very specialist group? Feeling doubtful this is going to work, I write something up anyway and send it across.

Ehsan receives it gratefully.

"You feeling better?" I add.

"Yeah, a little bit."

Small mercies. The day has felt like the first time in a long time that something has gone in the right direction. I sleep better that night than I have for weeks.

• • •

The next day (13 March) starts badly, as I wake up to read the news that the government has suspended community testing of possible coronavirus patients, to focus on hospitals. It seems that community spread has become accepted as inevitable. The day only gets worse from there. In the echo department, the patient with possible COVID from yesterday hasn't been tested and is still in the open bay. Clearly the message didn't get communicated. I text Piotr "What happened to the lady in bed 10?", but he doesn't respond. I think one of my colleagues, Flo, is covering the ward that week, so I message her directly. She comes straight back to me, saying "Let me look into it."

The department is mostly empty this morning, and Jack and I triage the requests as we did the day before. Today, there are far fewer, and generally only very urgent scans. Things are changing very rapidly now. Meanwhile, Dr Geffers messages me with: "Got a job for you." We have a quick phone call. He thinks that my idea about connecting with the most junior doctors in the hospital is a good idea and is delegating it back to me. I need to find out where they all are, who they are and if they have done all the PPE training.

I instantly realize that I don't actually know how many departments we have, let alone how to find out who is working there. Trying to be clever, I spend an hour going through WhatsApp groups and even phoning the medical education centre to see if they hold a list. They don't, though – only a list of the emails of all the doctors in the hospital, without any assigned department. Conscious I need to sort this today, I plough on, trying to build on an existing group of a swathe of the juniors. However, it quickly becomes apparent that at least two other people are trying to do the same job as me, and we've inevitably bumped into each other. A few fractious emails fly back and forth about who is supposed to be doing what. It's exhausting. We eventually decide that it'd be quicker for me to physically wander around and find people.

It's a big hospital and I end up essentially exploring it for the first time, going to wards and areas I have never been to before, finding a junior-looking person I've never met and signing them up to a new WhatsApp group, and asking them to invite their colleagues in the same department. It's surprisingly effective, and we set up a group by the afternoon. It quickly becomes apparent that the same confusion and frustration I was experiencing was nearly universal, but connecting and talking is really helpful, to avoid people going around the same circles many of us have looped through already. Initially it feels good, but it's clear that communications are going to be a problem if this is the effort required to physically connect with select staff groups in the hospital.

I write some of this feedback on one of the management groups, but it's met with stony silence. I then get an angry phone call from Dr Geffers, who has taken this as a criticism. Again, we go from fractious to fraternal over the course of the conversation.

"I just need something to do, I'm going crazy," I say.

"Wait till next week, you won't know what's hit you," Dr Geffers replies.

"That's exactly my point," I answer.

"There will be plenty to do, just wait."

But waiting is the one thing that we can't do. None of us can. I feel like I'm pulling my hair out.

Toward the end of the day Flo messages me: "Tests sent, patient in side room. Thanks." It seems curt. Perhaps it's been a crazy shift, as it so often is, but I'm just trying to help. I head home in a foul mood.

• • •

When I get back, Dilsan is watching the news. Overhead camera shots of Cheltenham Racecourse fill the screen, showing a sea of thousands of people around the track. Many are already calling for the cancellation of mass gatherings, and here is a huge and extremely packed gathering. The entire medical community has cancelled conferences for the whole summer, but the country continues to go its own way.

Boris Johnson and Chris Whitty conduct the daily press conference that evening, and there is some expectation that the government will announce some big intervention with regard to Cheltenham. They announce the cases (798) and the number of people who have already died (28), insisting they had "underlying health conditions", a phrase we have already heard over and over again until it has lost all meaning. After some explanatory remarks, they move on to questions, with clearly no plan to announce any large intervention. Is it the plan to actually let the virus run through the population? I ask myself. I can't understand how this plan tallies with all of the rest of the data about patients needing intensive care and becoming critically unwell. The phrase "we are following the science" comes up repeatedly.

"Do you think this is 'following the science'?" Dilsan asks.

"I think these decisions come from a very large committee and there will be another layer of politics and messaging over the top – to think these decisions are simple 'science' is a gross simplification. The numbers just don't add up," I say with a shrug.

"Beck said John is going to be on this evening," Dilsan reminds me, talking about my cousin's partner, Professor Edmunds, who's appearing on Channel 4 News again that evening. A phrase he uses sticks with me: "Without a vaccine, the only way out of the epidemic is herd immunity." He is right, given the fact that the virus cannot be controlled anymore, that we aren't testing in the community, and that by this time most countries in the world have confirmed cases, that there is only one way "out". But whatever the way "out" is, my overriding concern is the way "in" – how do we stop the virus from overwhelming the NHS, and how do we protect Ehsan and my dad?

Currently we look to be steamrolling ahead without significant government intervention, and the number of people infected by the virus continues to increase, reaching nearly

800 cases. Given that the incubation period from exposure to peak symptoms is reported as up to two weeks, and it would take two weeks to pull the proverbial brake after introducing lockdown measures, those 800 cases would be 10,000, and that's if we did something right now. Dilsan feels the same way, perhaps more so than me. She decides to message her extended family, the cousins she grew up with here in north London. She has been chatting to them more recently – it provides another insight into the wider world through the perspective of people from different walks of life; the general consensus among them is that there's nothing to worry about. Despite the jokes and the reminiscing, I can tell Dilsan is finding it incredibly frustrating. It feels like we are approaching a precipice. So, she decides to corral her cousins into a WhatsApp group, to connect and warn them, but I worry it'll do more harm than good and maybe descend into another source of frustration and division. She prepares a long and heavy message, outlining our concerns. Before she can send it to the group, one of her cousins, Jem, is too quick and messages the group as soon as he is added: "At last we will come together to fight this wild and dangerous creature." I can't help but laugh. Dilsan stays serious and tries to pull the conversation around to the gravity of the situation, to warn the group of what is likely coming. Her cousins listen, but the tone is light, and before long Dilsan is laughing at the decades-old private jokes only families have. It's good for her to connect.

I think of my own family and promise myself to call Mum and Dad tomorrow, to Skype with my brother Paul and his girls more. I also try and check in on our elderly neighbours.

As if on cue, an email lands in my inbox from my Aunt Judy. She has been planning her 80th birthday party for the end of the month, 26 March. A big family get-together is quite a rare and special occasion and this one has been in the works for nearly a year. My dad is one of eight brothers and sisters, and our extended family over the generations has grown to quite a large clan. But, all in their seventies and eighties now, my dad's generation are particularly vulnerable to COVID-19.

There has been some chatter over email for some time about what we should do about Aunt Judy's birthday party. I hadn't said anything as yet, for fear of being alarmist, but I think we are now beyond that. While Dilsan is connecting with her family, I'm advising my own to do the opposite. I try to do it as nicely as possible, pointing out that travelling by 26 March may be impossible anyway, but emphasizing that the risk of catching COVID-19 is high, given that people would need to come from all over the country. A crisis for the country on the scale of World War Two. While I feel somewhat relieved when my aunty responds, sad to cancel the party but under-standing of my reasons, it's also upsetting – my kids haven't even met many of their cousins and second cousins, and I was really looking forward to seeing them all together. I can't help wondering when it will be okay to get together again. Months from now? Years?

. . .

I seem to have fallen into a cycle of sleepless nights, followed by restless ones. Mercifully, the kids sleep through, but I find myself staring at the ceiling again at 5 a.m., flicking idly through news reports. I see that a director of one of the Lombardy medical schools has died from COVID-19. So many colleagues are losing their lives. What are we doing? I think angrily to myself. I creep downstairs to watch the sun rise and make a herbal tea. The sharp aroma of the peppermint and the warmth of the cup are life-giving.

Our family friend Sem messages me. She's terrified about her mum.

"Dom – I'm thinking about buying my mum a ventilator. Just as a precaution."

We use a variety of devices to physically get air into a human being who is struggling to breathe; we divide them into invasive devices, which require the insertion of a physical tube into the mouth or through a hole in the neck, and non-invasive devices, which are masks that are worn or strapped to the mouth and nose (or sometimes just the nose) and blast pressurized oxygen into a patient. These devices have various settings, with the highest-end invasive ventilators being able to control all sorts of parameters of breathing, including the pressure at rest and the pressure inhaled, the oxygen concentration, the rate and rhythm of breathing, including augmenting the patient's breathing or simply breathing for them, and being able to switch automatically through all of this, if needed. These are typically what we in the medical world would refer to as "ventilators" – the machines you see in intensive care, which provide long-term ventilation typically over a period of days or weeks. The settings on these machines are slowly adjusted over time to help the patients get back to breathing for themselves, a process called weaning. We also use ventilators during surgeries, but these are less subtle devices, generally, only intended for use in the short term and without the range of modes that we can get in intensive care. The non-invasive devices are simpler still, capable of controlling the pressure at rest and on inspiration, or simply blowing very high volumes of oxygen at high pressure up the nose.

It's not clear which "ventilator" the news cycle has been referring to, but it has clearly affected Sem. What exactly is meant by a "home ventilator", I don't know. In rare cases, some patients could have proper invasive ventilation at home, supplied through a hole in the neck created by a procedure called a tracheostomy. But this requires incredibly complex care, of the ventilator, the airway and the patient. The subject of home ventilation inspired heated debated on our social media when this popped up in the morning's headlines a few days ago.

I explain as much to Sem.

"Dude – what else can I do?" comes the reply.

The only thing her mum can realistically do, given that she's immunosuppressed with lung disease and has had a previous heart attack, is to stay at home. Just as with Ehsan, I suggest that she self-isolates, and that everybody stays away as much as possible.

"Do you mean actually not leave the house at all?" she asks.

"Yes. That's what Ehsan is doing."

"Wow. So, it's that bad?"

"Yes." I add a link to the *Independent* article I wrote. "This is worth reading," I say.

A few minutes passes while she reads it. "Unbelievable, I'm taking Emma out of nursery," she writes back.

"Lots of people are. Kids, thank God, don't seem to get sick, though. Not properly sick, anyway."

"Thank God. Call me later," Sem signs off.

"Sure," I say.

Dilsan comes downstairs to find me, but the kids haven't emerged yet. It's a very rare moment for us these days. We sit on the couch with tea, enjoying the peace. Dilsan passes me her phone, showing me the chat on her cousins' WhatsApp group.

"What do you reckon about this?" she says.

Dilsan's cousin is telling the group that a nurse who lives a road over from her was found dead at home. I'm sceptical, as it sounds like a third- or fourth-hand account.

"There would be news of that, no?" I say.

"Would there?" Dilsan asks.

I don't really know the answer to that question, I suppose. It seems rumours are everywhere, like the story I hear about the intensive care department containing three ITU consultants with COVID being kept alive on ventilators. The name of the hospital changes each time I read it. Then a friend texts me and asks if it's true that we have two registrars on our unit at the moment. It's the same rumour I've heard about his hospital. The medical airwaves are clotted with information and misinformation.

Meanwhile, the guidelines for masks have just changed. For both positive cases and suspected cases, we should be wearing a simple surgical mask instead of the full PPE we have been using. I'm getting messages from some of the junior doctors, unable to find a mask that they fit tested with. It seems clear that the guidance has only changed because we couldn't hope to supply full PPE for every front-facing member of staff. With a head full of both rumours and facts about colleagues falling ill, I reach out to another group of campaigners. We need to do something about this, I think, but Dilsan is less convinced that we can do anything, that we should do anything. Ayla interrupts our conversation by waking up in her usual way, by shouting "I want dinner!" very loudly from her room.

We have a normal day and go to the park, leaving our phones at home. The day is bright and cold, with barely a breeze. We get ice cream and coffee and wander up and down the length of the small stream. Ayla spends too much time on the swings, while Zach nods off in the buggy. Sitting there, watching kids barrel up and down the playground while their parents quietly chat and couples walk their dogs, it seems like life is simply carrying on. But it doesn't feel real – it feels insulated from what's happening in the world we see through our television and phone screens. In that moment, it feels easy to simply choose what to believe, and to ignore everything else.

We could simply do nothing. Life is full as it is – we can weather COVID-19 at home, get on with the work in front of us and hope for the best. We'll do what we can for the loved ones around us, and that will be enough. Breathing in the cold spring air, giving up this clenched fist of worry in my chest, brings relief. I feel lighter. We nip by the shops on the way home, make Ayla's favourite dinner of spaghetti and meatballs, put the kids to bed and watch a movie. No news, no phones. It feels nice.

· · ·

The next morning, Sunday 15 March, I wake up at 6 a.m. to find the bed empty. Zach has just woken up, so I go and fetch him and steal downstairs to find Dilsan. She's pacing around the kitchen, talking animatedly on the phone.

"It's going to be a shitshow. I don't know why they aren't locking down. We should do something."

"Who is it?" I mouth, juggling Zach in one arm while making his breakfast in the other.

"It's Nej," Dilsan whispers. Nej is Dilsan's cousin, a senior banking executive and someone whose judgement both Dilsan and I trust implicitly. "Yeah, Dom's up… he says hi… okay, I'll speak to him. Thanks, Nej." Dilsan hangs up.

"What's going on, my love?" I ask.

"We need to do something, something to get the government to lock down. Nej has been lobbying his daughter's school to close already."

This is a decided turnaround from where we landed yesterday, but trying to do something is a better channel for all this nervous energy than letting it burn us up.

"I was telling Nej about the herd immunity stuff, about the exponential cases. He wants to help."

"What do you propose?" I ask, thinking about the role reversal, given that it's normally me that's running the campaigning ideas up the flagpole.

"What about some sort of letter to the government?" Dilsan says.

I consider this. We have done similar things before, although not for years. A few years ago, I made videos about the NHS to try to educate and inspire people to support what

I still believe is our greatest and most humane institution. I have a few connections in various campaign groups that might be able to help. Dilsan has her social connections as well. Via a few of my threads I've had some journalists reach out on email and Twitter – maybe we could try to land the letter somewhere there.

"Okay. Where do we start?" I say.

We try to find a whiteboard, sure that we used to have one in the kids' room or something. But we can only find the markers for it. We realize our cupboards are made of the same material, albeit slightly off-white, so we use one to start drawing up a list of points for the letter, who to get it to, timescales. I reach out to a campaign group for the NHS for help, and the response is immediate and forceful, with tens of professionals keen to get involved. They have a dedicated press officer who helps us guide the letter. In the midst of this, I tweet a thread with my numbers on ventilator capacity, about where the "NHS capacity" line should be to flatten the curve beneath it. By lunchtime our cupboards are covered in a spidery scrawl of ideas, facts and figures. The letter we draft reads:

> The NHS on whose frontlines we work is an outlier in the international community. Unlike our colleagues across the world, we are being instructed to refuse World Health Organization advice of strict social distancing and rigorous community testing. Instead, we are adopting a strategy with a disturbing lack of evidence or detail to it, one whose reckless pursuit will result in enormous and unnecessary loss of life.

The government's "herd immunity" strategy takes no account of the finite capacity of our healthcare system. According to leaked documents, it presumes an 80 per cent infection rate, which would require ten times as many ventilators as we have, and at least double the beds. Nor is it scientifically validated: we do not know whether coronavirus infection can even confer immunity.

The NHS is not ready for the crisis the government is about to allow to occur. We must therefore buy time with aggressive containment measures, including banning mass gatherings, closing the schools, isolating the vulnerable and restricting travel.

With an incubation period of two weeks, any action we take now won't have an effect for a fortnight. We need to act today – better yet, two weeks ago.

It's an iterative process, but we get there in the end. Dilsan posts it on her groups and I ask my groups to share and sign it – in an hour, we have nearly 500 NHS staff signatures. We order some food, and over dinner, I check the news for that day. Many groups are now pulling in the same direction, and behavioural scientists have called out the lack of a decision to lock down as being based on "flawed science". Richard Horton, editor of *The Lancet* (the peer-reviewed medical journal), has called for a drastic change in direction. It seems like public pressure is mounting. Also, a boss of mine and a good friend of a friend, Dr Matt Webb, messages me about the internal planning at his hospital, highlighting an issue I haven't even considered: the oxygen supply. Although nearly every hospital bed will have a port for oxygen to be supplied, not all the vents can be used at the same time, raising the very real possibility that in a hospital full of respiratory patients, suddenly we could run out of oxygen. Thanking him for the heads-up, I add the detail to our notes.

Buoyed by the support, we plough on, and manage to get the letter into the *Independent* for publication the next day, supported by over 1,000 signatures from NHS staff. Sam, the press officer from Keep Our NHS Public (KONP), has managed to secure some media coverage for tomorrow and is pushing me to go on TV. I've only been on television once before, on a local station broadcast, but I didn't think much of my voice or appearance. I've stuck to print ever since (with the exception of the video explainer I did back in the first week of March for the Press Association), even subtitling a video animation I made about the NHS rather than record a voiceover for it. I also have to think of the ramifications at work – it's very possible that by making a visible and controversial statement, even one that might ultimately save lives, I will lose my job. But I begin to suspect it will be worth it.

A friend of mine, Rita, gives me some really useful advice about how to use the very short minutes of time to the maximum, how to deal with questions and stick to the points. We run the arguments by Nej, who is used to high-powered presentations and making an impact with large organizations. He offers me some pointers and helps us get the wording right; I even scribble a few of his phrases down in my notebook. Sam has actually lined up a radio interview that night, and then television coverage in the early morning, to fit around my working hours.

The radio was a good warm-up – I could have my notes in front of me and could read the writing on the cupboard doors in my kitchen at the same time. Nej and a few others listened in. I stumbled a bit, didn't quite manage to close out everything I wanted to say, but got across what I could the best I could. Nej had some great feedback and so did Dilsan. I wrote it down, and we refined some points and phrases. The *Independent* confirmed that the letter would be going out tomorrow. We were ready. I went to sleep nervous but determined. Time to spark off.

• • •

The next morning, I wake at 5 a.m., get dressed quietly and leave deliberately early to make sure I'm not late. I walk to the station to go over my notes on my phone, trying to get the first few points memorized so I won't stumble on them. Already feeling quite sick with nerves, my morning coffee makes it worse, and I can't seem to focus. I try to write down a few answers to potentially challenging questions: Who are you to say this? Why shouldn't we trust Chris Whitty? What is the way out of this? I use the tidbits that Rita taught me, like the technique "accept, bridge, counter" (ABC). But trying to remember the answers feels like trying to hold water in my hands. Tube station after station flies by too quickly, and I'm distracted enough to miss my connection to Westminster. My head is jumbled – I feel like I'm going to mess this up, when the stakes are so high already.

I pop out of the tube station and struggle to find the interview location. Sky have banned visitors to the studio, especially medical staff working with confirmed or possible cases, so they have set up an area outside Westminster gardens. Not really knowing the area, it takes me a while to find the spot, but even then, I'm half an hour early. The crew sends me to find a coffee and come back. I get lost, then they call me to get me back earlier than initially planned. So, despite the preparation, I find myself madly sprinting back to where I started, just in time to get positioned and then bam. I'm speaking live on Sky News. Without being able to see the interviewer – there's just a voice in my ear – I try to give the lines I've memorized directly to the camera. I don't know what to do with my hands, and they migrate all around me as I talk and try to answer the questions. We talk about the lack of PPE equipment, and the fact that additional ventilators are only now being ordered, the potential to run out of oxygen and intensive care beds already, the WHO and Richard Horton of *The Lancet*. I don't mess up majorly, I hope. And just like that, it's over, the crew usher me away and I wander off, to get to work on time.

Nerves settled, I pop into a coffee shop, order a flat white and text Dilsan. She is proud. Nej has some comments and says I should call him later. The barista sees me eyeing the pastries and asks if I want one.

"F**k it, the world is ending, sure, give me one." It's a pretty accurate summary of how I've been feeling for the last few days.

The barista looks askance at me.

"Do you want two?" she asks. It sounds absurd. It all is, I suppose.

"It's not that bad," I joke, and pay for the coffee and pastry.

I sip on my drink before I pull my mask back on and head off down to the tube again to go to work.

• • •

Back in the echo department again that day, it's essentially a ghost town. There are very few patients to scan, and I try to work on my logbook. There is a general anxiety and confusion about what protection staff should and shouldn't be wearing to scan patients. Jack has brought in a whole bunch of industrial masks his mum sent him. Other departments are doing different things, and we've already heard stories of senior management getting involved, asking staff to remove masks being worn against policy. I'm not sure what the best solution is – staff need to feel safe, but equally, resources are tight and the whole place feels only a spark away from mass panic. All of this would be mitigated if we'd only had more time to prepare going forward; at least our campaign is doing something to address that, though.

Glancing at my phone, I have a few random texts from colleagues and family I haven't spoken to for months. It feels good to be doing something – it's calming and purposeful. I catch up with Nej at lunchtime. He gives me some good feedback and we try to sharpen things a bit more. Although we are from very different worlds, there's a mutual respect that makes our partnership work well. A reminder email pops into my inbox offering heavily discounted will-making services for NHS staff. I give the company a call back – the customer services agent is sympathetic, and it's far cheaper than I was expecting.

We go through the process and then arrange a follow-up with their legal team later in the week.

The afternoon slides by and finishes early, due to a combination of fewer appointments booked in and fewer patients turning up to their appointments. Before I know it, I'm haring across London again, this time heading to Oxford Circus, and the BBC. I've walked past this building many times in the past, but never crossed the threshold. The semi-circular design feels imposing as I walk past its wings. I feel a bit sick but try to remember the talking points I went over this morning. I feel incredibly self-conscious entering the lobby, with its 20-foot screen streaming BBC News live, and groups of harassed and important-looking people moving back and forth from the entrance. The place feels alive. I give my name to the receptionist, for Hugh Pym, the Health Editor for BBC News. I take a seat on a trendy but very uncomfortable sofa and flick idly through my phone while I wait.

I've never seen Hugh standing up in real life before, only ever sitting down or on his profile on Twitter. He's imposingly tall, and older than I expect, with wings of white framing a kindly face and a few laughter lines creasing his eyes. We don't shake hands, but have an affable chat while the crew set up a spot outside the main studio. The questions are the same as before, but the interview is a lot longer and I end up in unplanned territory.

"Are you and your colleagues worried about the pandemic?" Hugh asks me.

"Um…." I think of Jack with his home-made masks, and Nat worried about her kids, and all the other dozens of conversations we've been having for the last few weeks. "I'm making a will this week. I suppose that about sums it up."

Hugh is genuinely taken aback. "That's a bit strong. Can we do that again?" he asks.

The whole interview takes 20 minutes, and then there's some downtime while the crew take some technical shots where Hugh and I chat, off the record. I'm shocked by how much of a surprise this has come to even the journalists covering the story – the rapidity of the pandemic, the need for lockdown, the lack of preparedness. I think Hugh is genuinely rattled. I need to remember that everybody is experiencing this as a normal person first, even journalists.

"Don't you trust Chris Whitty?" Hugh asks me (as I imagined he might).

"I think he's the best possible person for the job right now, but to think his decisions are being taken in isolation is naive, in my opinion." Hugh thanks me and I head off again, reflecting on how everyone is transitioning slowly to accepting the scale of the crisis. It's a relief in many ways, as it becomes increasingly evident that our concerns weren't hysterical at all, and are now being vindicated.

I catch up with Dilsan on the phone, conveying that hopefully some of the interview will make it into the news at 6 p.m. I head to a nearby Pizza Express for an early dinner while I'm waiting to appear as a guest on Channel 4 News. A TV in the restaurant is showing the COVID press conference and the language has changed significantly. Boris Johnson announces measures to reduce social contact, although the language is woolly and seems to be heavily couched in advice – advice to avoid pubs and restaurants and to work from home if you can, and advice that emergency workers won't support mass gatherings, but no direct bans or enforcements or support announced. "Shielding" of highly vulnerable adults is announced for a few days' time, although I'm not sure why the further delay. Boris has appeared to cave to pressure from Scotland and Wales, by following suit and announcing the closure of schools for all children except key workers. At least Ehsan now has some clear guidance on what he should be doing and so will the school. It's not without irony that I watch Boris advise that people avoid pubs and restaurants while I'm sitting in Pizza Express. As last meals out go, I reflect, this isn't a bad one, if a little lonely. I wonder when I will come back to dining out again.

The measures imposed seem like a step in the right direction, but it's not nearly far enough. I wonder, why the change now? Dilsan is watching, and calls me.

"Are you watching the press conference?"

"It's good news, isn't it?"

"Seems a bit woolly – what is actually going to change? Everything's still open."

"Mmm. This is true. But at least we are pushing on an open door now."

"Okay, my love. Didn't see you on BBC News."

"Think they cut out most of it in the end, I suppose because of the press conference."

"Never mind. What time is Channel 4?"

"8 p.m., I think."

"How are you feeling?"

To be honest, I'm shattered. A manic, sleepless 48 hours, followed by a day traipsing all over London. "All good. Gonna have a quick coffee."

She rings off.

Another journalist messages me over Twitter, although not in a professional capacity but a personal one. She has seen the news and is worried for her own health, having moderate-severe asthma. I try and find some resources for her, but information is still pretty sparse. I send what I can find on the government and NHS websites, and a few screen grabs from asthma societies in the UK and the US. She is grateful.

So many young and vulnerable people are staring down the barrel of self-isolation for weeks if not months. Ehsan and Nesli are chatting on our family group, trying to work out how he can shield for 12 weeks with two kids in nursery and Nesli still teaching. Now there's official guidance, some of the plans we've already discussed would be easier to sort. We agree to have a chat about it tomorrow.

I've got some time to get across to the last stop of the night, a satellite studio for Channel 4, as they want me to stay isolated from the panel. I decide to walk. Night has well and truly set in, and Oxford Street is eerily quiet. A homeless man is laughing and shouting at one end of a bus stop, while a small group of people give him a wide berth at the other end. What will happen to him? Without a place to go, how can anyone without a home lock down? The night is far chillier than the day, and I pull my coat closer as I walk on. A few minutes down the street, I hear the soaring strings of a busking violinist outside Debenhams. His music is bittersweet and haunting, all the more so playing to a nearly deserted street, with buses flashing by. Thinking of my sister, I fear that musicians are going to really struggle with this new world. We all are, I suppose, in all our different ways.

By the time I get to the Channel 4 studio, I'm yawning hungrily, and my face aches with tiredness. The cold has really hit me hard on top of an already exhausting day. There's some confusion about who is supposed to get me to the right place, and it takes a while to solve, as the broadcast time gets closer and closer. With just a few minutes to spare, someone escorts me to a broom-cupboard-sized room with padded walls and a green screen. The room reminds me of a hostage video: a single chair, a single camera, a microphone on the floor. I can't hear or see anything else, other than a feed of the sound from Channel 4. A crackly voice breaks the newscast.

"Can you not slouch so much? We need to align the shot."

Embarrassed, I sit up in the chair, attempting to rearrange my outfit. I try to catch my reflection in the camera lens, but then wish I hadn't been reminded of my beardless face and too-long hamster haircut. And then it's too late to worry about that, because Jon Snow is introducing the panel, Professor Karol Sikora, an oncologist and the dean of the country's only private medical school (at the University of Buckingham), Dr Bharat Pankhania, a public health lecturer, and me, an idiot with Google and a napkin, and a big mouth. I try to stick to the narrative as I remember it as best I can. They move on to Professor Sikora, who suggests "everything is under control" and makes a comment about avoiding "draconian" measures. Assuming I'm not on camera, I don't take much care with my reaction and rub my eyes with the characteristic frustration of the tired. Even now, the idea of locking people away doesn't seem palatable, although the government could do a lot more to make it work, given the time. Dr Pankhania, the public health expert, outlines the same position supporting our letter. It's remarkable to hear so much expertise that up until now was dismissed, as the government claimed to be following "THE science". The interview comes to a close, but I'm not sure what is still live and isn't, so I sit there awkwardly for a number of minutes. Eventually one of the technicians comes and lets me out.

They call me a car, and just as quickly, the interview and this crazy day are both over, and I head home. I speak to Nej, who is very pleased. Dilsan is proud. Ayla asks, "When will Daddy be on PAW Patrol?", which is the only television appearance my daughter respects. It may very well be that we did nothing, helped no one; the government was always going to introduce a soft lockdown today, and would pay no heed to anything any other group said. But if there is even a remote possibility that someone watching took the guidance seriously when they otherwise wouldn't, or shielded a loved one, or took steps to prepare, then, whatever the fall-out, it will have been worth it. At least we tried.

CHAPTER 6

Complications

That night, Dilsan and I sleep better than we have done for weeks. Like a coiled spring, however, the COVID cases have built up for weeks, and now we have to deal with that explosive energy being released into London and the rest of the country. The news this morning is full of the government's U-turn on the lockdown since yesterday (16 March), citing a "change in the science" and a report from the Imperial SAGE group that suggests the NHS won't be able to cope without an immediate lockdown, exactly as we were saying only a day ago. I'm not sure where the "science" has changed, but at least increasingly we are all on the same page.

Given this change in the government's messaging from no lockdown measures to at least softly advocating for people to stay at home if they can, I'm expecting the morning commute to be blissfully empty, but it seems just as busy as ever. I have to change at Finsbury Park and the platform is packed. Without clear and firm messaging and with little support to make any drastic changes, people are unlikely to instantly abandon their daily lives and livelihoods, I suppose. I try to keep my head down and stick to the corners of the tube carriages, my nose buried in my Twitter feed. I see lots of supportive comments, and lots of negative ones too, branding me an "alarmist", an "opportunist" and "self-promoting" after my performance on TV the night before. It's unsurprising, but after the emotional and physical strain of the past few days, the attacks, from colleagues especially, get to me more than they should. The uncertainty is causing tension, and opinions and feelings are riding high. I get it. But then a comment under one tweet catches my eye:

"I want to thank you again because you kindly put together a thread about two and a half weeks back, a summary of how to prepare behaviourally and practically. I was able to absorb, adjust and also share that vital info with my family/circles. It was simple and very important."

It's such a short message, but something inside me snaps. I find myself sitting on the tube silently in tears. It has released something and I feel so much better for it. Being the guy on the train carriage crying to himself also helps my social distancing no end. A few days ago, I wrote down some simple rules for staying mentally balanced during the pandemic, and "having a good cry now and then" was number 1. Exercise was number 2, and "accepting it's okay to not be okay" was number 3. I write a quick note about what I might need and what other NHS workers will require in the next few weeks during the lockdown: food (with supermarkets reducing hours and local restaurants closing), counselling services, help with childcare and bereavement support.

We've moved over entirely to telephone clinics now, and the department is empty when I arrive. We are still physically manning the clinic rooms just in case a patient doesn't get the message and turns up, or needs to be seen in the flesh, though. There's no consultant, but a list as usual, featuring the same appointment slots and patient notes – the only difference is there are no physical people to see. I pull up the first patient's notes, sipping on a coffee. It's all very civilized.

Trina is a 75-year-old retired chemist. Her heart function has deteriorated over the past several years, although it's not clear why from her notes; her heart arteries are normal and an MRI of the heart tissue doesn't reveal any specific diagnosis, only that instead of a thick fist of beating muscle, her heart is thinned and ballooned, like a canvas bag of blood. When I click the little "play" icon, the grey-and-white heart barely moves, each beat just registering as a shiver. Trina is on a cocktail of medicines already, and has had a special pacemaker fitted to make her heart beat more efficiently. She has a likely genetic heart condition and is on good medication already without experiencing any symptoms, so there isn't much to optimize. I dial her number but there's no answer. I don't really know the protocol now – perhaps that counts as a Did Not Attend?

I move on to the next patient, thinking I'll come back to Trina. Harriet is also 75 years old; she's a retired architect with a swollen foot. Her GP is convinced that her foot is caused by a failing heart and would like her to be seen. She's already had some blood tests and a heart scan, which were all normal. Hoping this will be a straightforward consultation, I try Harriet, but there's no answer. There's a mobile number on the file, which I try too, but it goes straight to voicemail. Although she has now missed two appointments, I give Harriet the benefit of the doubt and leave the clinic extension number on the voicemail.

I try Trina again – this time the phone rings three times and is picked up by a baritone male voice.

"Hello?"

"Hello, I'm looking for Trina Augustine?" I say.

"Who is this?" comes the reply.

This is tricky – I can't say who I am without announcing that this is a doctor's appointment, which could breach Trina's confidentiality. Equally, I can't ask Trina's permission to let that be known if she doesn't get to the phone.

"I can't say – could I speak to Trina?"

"She can't talk right now, she's waiting for the doctor to call," comes the reply from who I now assume is Trina's son.

"That's me!" I cut in, feeling I'm about to be hung up on.

"Ah. Why didn't you just say so?" he says slightly irritably, before I hear "Mum – it's the doctor" spoken louder.

Thankfully, this is a telephone appointment and my eye rolling isn't visible.

"Hello, doctor – how are you today?" comes a cheery Caribbean accent, so bright that it brings a smile to me as well.

"Very good, Trina, how are you?" As we chat, I can search through her records as needed, going back and forth and making notes on drugs and other medical conditions.

We go through the usual questions.

"How's your breathing?" I ask.

"No trouble at all, doctor," Trina answers.

"How far can you walk before you feel breathless?"

"Oh, miles and miles."

"And how's your weight?"

"Oh, I don't know… hang on," she says. Then there's a clunk, which I guess is the sound of Trina putting the phone down while she goes and weighs herself, leaving me listening to silence and waiting. The novelty of being made to wait on the patient makes me smile again. After about a minute, she comes back to the phone, slightly breathless.

"It's good," Trina says.

I nearly laugh out loud at that.

"And did you get a figure from the scale, Trina?"

"Oh… hold on." There's another clunk. I'm genuinely quite enjoying this.

"It's 85 kg," comes the eventual answer. I check our last weight on the system: it's 87 kg. Great. We rattle through the rest of the questions. At the end, Trina has one for me.

"Can we do this again next time? We are in Streatham and it's a long way into the hospital there."

I check the time – this whole consultation has only taken five minutes, and we've covered all the bases. I really don't think we would have done anything differently if Trina had been here in person.

"Yes, of course," I say.

I book a follow-up appointment for her, along with a separate appointment to check her pacemaker. Trina jots down the dates in her diary.

"Thank you, doctor."

"Take care," I say.

As I hang up, the phone rings again straight away, and it's Harriet returning my phone call. And the clinic is away! I rattle through the list in two-thirds of the usual time. Only one or two patients aren't contactable, and every single one seems genuinely happy to be called at home. I can't help but think that this is the future.

I finish up with the last patient at 11 a.m. The clinic is done, an hour early. I have a free afternoon to catch up on some admin back home. The kids will be overjoyed, although I suspect that might dampen my chances of actually getting anything done.

• • •

On the way home I check my messages – I have an email from an anaesthetic consultant called Michelle Dawson. The message is entitled "PPE". It's short and simply reads "I have a contact that can get 30 million FFP3* masks here in a month, but the government won't go outside the normal supply chain. Thinking of speaking to the media – can you help?" I fire back a response immediately and we exchange mobile numbers. As I step off the bus into a bright, sunny March afternoon, my phone rings.

"Hi, Dom. This is Michelle," comes a bright, Northern accent.

"Hi, Michelle. Thanks for getting in touch."

"For 10 years, I've been clinical lead in charge of procurement at my hospital and have a contact that can supply 30 million masks directly from China."

"Wow, Michelle, that's massive news. How can we get this going?"

---

* FFP standing for Filtering Facepiece Respirator, with the "3" denoting the highest of the three classes of filtering efficiency

"Oh, that's not all. My contact is also working on a vaccine, but the government fund has already run out for vaccine manufacturing."

"What do you mean... run out?" I answer, disbelievingly.

"They allocated £20 million, which has all gone. The vaccine is eligible for funding but there was no more budgeted," Michelle tells me.

"This is crazy, Michelle. How did you get involved?"

"Oh, I just had a few days off and thought I'd try to help," she says.

I'm bowled over by Michelle: by her humility, drive, and practical determination.

I don't know how I can help, really, but I offer to connect her to a journalist, imagining that perhaps they can brief on the story and put some pressure on the government. I leave them to it, wondering what might come of it.

I get home when the sun is still shining, at the witching hour for children: 4 p.m. They're hungry, restless and hysterical, but with both Dilsan and me at home, we can all roll around, splash through bath-time and then the kids are thoroughly knocked out in time for bed. At 6.30 p.m., with both kids asleep, Dilsan and I have a glass of cold white wine. The contrast between this moment of blissful peace and the chaos of just a few minutes ago is remarkable. We sit and chat in the kitchen and I fill her in about the call with Michelle.

"That's amazing news," Dilsan says.

"Yes, I need to check on what happened with that. I would think it might be quite difficult to get that off the ground."

"She's just doing something this massive, on her day off?"

"Yeah – it's incredible, really."

"Everyone wants to help, I guess."

That's true. All that pent-up energy – the anxiety, the tension – has to go somewhere; everyone must be feeling the same, now, as a nation.

That evening, an email lands in my inbox from our rota coordinators. We are establishing new rotas daily to keep up with the rapidly rising number of cases, and they are now asking if any of us cardiology registrars have intensive care experience. As a group, most of us have done at least a little time there, and a lot more visiting the unit to see sick patients and for consults. I reply, happy to help with whatever, and book into the intensive care training scheduled for the following week. I suppose we are going to all transition into ICU eventually.

Dilsan is worried, though, when I tell her.

"Do you think it's a good idea? Aren't you going to be more exposed?" she asks.

I wonder if that's true, actually – yes, that's where a lot of the higher-risk special procedures occur, generating the very fine particles of virus that can hang around in air for up to three hours, but all staff wear full personal protective equipment at all times around those patients. I'm not sure of the answer, really. Certainly, the rumours are still flying around about anaesthetists becoming unwell, and other staff, such as ENT (ear, nose and throat) surgeons, being admitted to intensive care themselves. In my heart of hearts, I know it will be fine, but I can't seem to put that into words that Dilsan's surgical-clinical brain will accept. In the end, there's no objectivity to it. Just a bit of pragmatism and a bit of faith, I suppose.

"What will be will be. I think it'll be fine. And there isn't much choice, anyway," I answer her.

After the last few weeks of ramping tension, like a roller coaster cranking to its peak, it feels like we are over the hump, our course is now locked, and we are hurtling downwards. I find it hard to sleep that night, the events of the day churning and mixing in my mind: the phone calls from the hospital, Michelle, the plan for working in intensive care next week. There's something about Michelle's "we can do this ourselves" attitude that I can't let go of. We will all need something to focus that energy into over the coming weeks and months – I will have work, but what about Dilsan? When the lockdown comes, that'll be her freedom gone, so newly earned after nine months of maternity leave already. If she gets called up from maternity early, back to her surgical job, I'm not sure how we will cope at all.

The phrase "everyone wants to help" keeps turning around in my brain, like a crossword clue that I can't seem to place yet. And then, somewhere in that limbo between sleep and wakefulness at 2 a.m., an idea pops into my head nearly fully formed. The idea is to start a charity that can do all the things Michelle is trying to do, and hopefully more. To provide all the things we NHS workers might need in the coming weeks. In the long term, it might be able to support the families of those that might lose their lives – the kind of things that I would want for Ayla and Zach if the worst should happen.

Above all, I want to try and make the most of the energy and goodwill that's out there for the NHS right now, that common desire to help. The times are radical, and a radical energy possesses us all, an energy to be saddled and harnessed. If this was indeed, as people are referring to it, a war, then the frontline would be the hospitals and GP surgeries. Yet, none of us are soldiers – we didn't sign up to be in the firing line – so no one's prepared and many of us need help.

Dilsan finds me at 5 a.m., scrawling through PowerPoint slides, huddled in a blanket.

"Dom, are you okay?"

She looks genuinely worried, wondering if the stressors of the last few days have finally caused something to snap.

"I'm good. Really," I answer. "Have a look at this," I say, swinging the laptop toward her. My head feels clearer than it has done for some time. "We should start a charity."

She doesn't look any less worried.

"No, really. It's okay. Everyone is going to want to help, and we are going to need it. A charity to protect everything about NHS workers – their physical and mental health – now and long into the future."

"But this kind of stuff takes months or years to set up," Dilsan says, intrigued but sceptical. Through bleary eyes I note the time is still only just after 5 a.m. I can't really blame her.

"We can do it fast – COVID causes are already getting fast-tracked. Look, these are our values: speed, trust, 0 per cent bullshit. We'll just raise money and get stuff direct to our colleagues."

Dilsan pauses.

"I like it," she says, becoming more convinced. "What kind of stuff?"

Over a cup of tea, we go over what the charity is and what it might be, and form a plan together.

Supplying personal protective equipment – the visors, masks, gown and gloves – is going to be an incredibly difficult issue. With the government so underprepared, and already key supplies, such as the different mask types we use, running out where I work, the situation is only going to deteriorate. My plan is to buy it, make it and push the government to get it – if we are going to protect healthcare workers, we have to start here.

As the restaurants and shops begin to close after lockdown, food is becoming increasingly scarce. I've already found that many of the shops around my hospital are closing early, and, on the weekends, it is impossible to access food sometimes. I am now genuinely worried about getting through the day. The shelves have already been bare for days, and only Iceland thus far has made any allowances for the elderly. Perhaps we could get food to NHS workers, or maybe create online deliveries for them, or secure special time slots for them in supermarkets. I have experienced first-hand the unfettered joy of a surprise pizza or takeaway in the middle of a difficult shift. How uplifting those small tokens can be.

Childcare is already a major issue and is turning into a nightmare. Nurseries are already reducing hours, and surely will close soon. Many medics on long shifts rely on after-school clubs and pre-school drop-offs, and a lot of us are already utilizing elderly grandparents to cover the gaps, which poses another significant risk. How will we be able to adapt? Dilsan and I have been keeping Ayla out of nursery for a few days already. We might be able to scrape by, with Beck helping and Dilsan on maternity still. We had hoped to try to find a nanny in time for Dilsan to return to work. The charity will need to help those struggling to look after their kids and keep their shifts.

Then there was mental health. Dilsan and I have already talked about our own mental states and how we could try to stay sane in lockdown. Hunched over a cup of tea as the dawn sun breaches the horizon, struggling to think clearly, counselling and support services seem particularly poignant. There's no point getting through the pandemic physically intact and emerging mentally broken. We are thinking about us and our kids, but also the million-plus healthcare workers out there facing potentially their worst ever time at work and at home. We decide that counselling will be key to anything we do.

Lastly, for all the above reasons, we could raise money to help pay for the vital things that healthcare workers could need help with to get through – transport, accommodation, childcare and food. Anything that makes NHS workers' lives easier or safer in this time, we want to do. We want to connect the public goodwill to help the NHS. To help them help us.

I show her the name I've come up with: Healthcare Extraordinary Response Organisation and Support.

"Heross?"

"Yes. No. *Heroes*. It's an acronym."

"But it's spelt wrong."

"Oh yeah, you're right. Let me think about that. So, what do you think of the plan?"

Dilsan looks at me levelly.

"Love the idea. Not keen on the name."

"Oh, really?"

"Dom – do you consider yourself a hero?"

"Obviously not."

"Well, neither do I, and neither do any of the people we work with." Dilsan pauses.

"It doesn't necessarily refer to healthcare workers – it could apply to anyone going the extra mile in the pandemic. Something to tap into that energy to do more in an emergency, I suppose."

"Mmm… I still don't like it," Dilsan replies.

"Anyway, it's an acronym. I'm sure we won't even use it that much."

I come to eat these words, on a daily basis.

"So, are we doing this?"

Dilsan smiles and rubs my head. "Do you really need to ask?" she says.

She sips her tea, and an idea occurs to her.

"Do you know who would be really into this? Nej."

It's only just past 6 a.m. so we resist the compulsion to ring him at once. We decide to call him later, and I don't have a shift today, so no big rush. As the sun rises clear of the trees, the world is waking up, and it's a world on fire. My WhatsApp doctor groups buzz angrily with testimonials from all over London; there are no alcohol wipes anywhere in the hospital so the on-call pager has been wrapped inside a glove and a plastic baggy with an apologetic note. We argue even now over the strategy the government has taken, and more than a few doctors decide to leave groups, presumably because they simply haven't got the headspace for it. The tension is running so high, it's almost audible. It reads like a hundred little fires, burning all over the capital; several hospitals have run out of masks, and some doctors have been issued their own to guard jealously while on call. Managers are running down corridors to urgently solve problems. Northwick Park Hospital in north-west London has declared a critical incident as it has run out of beds, has had to convert operating theatres for intensive care patients and is overflowing to nearby units. To put it mildly, one of my friends, a fellow medic, writes, "this is all getting a little out of hand".

"Meltdown" has arrived, right on schedule. But no one can believe how this seems to have happened in a single day. Just yesterday, a consultant from Northwick Park was reassuring the public, and now we are overwhelmed. Our Facebook groups seethe and boil with reports of hundreds of COVID cases at hospitals already and rumours that a registrar has died at an intensive care unit in London. Some of the medics with older children are very worried about the schools staying open for their children, forcing them to go in and possibly be exposed to other children. This dark red wall of anger and frustration is penetrated by small glimmers of light: already a group of medical students is offering to provide key workers with childcare; a PDF file providing COVID management tips is jumping from group to group; and daily briefings are being set up at some hospitals to help keep staff up to date and informed. Some places seem to be ahead of the curve, arranging video teleconferences, closing clinics and practising social distancing. Other hospitals appear to be way behind, cramming all their staff into a single lecture theatre (where social distancing just isn't possible) to make announcements, keeping clinics open, and even castigating staff for sending too many swabs to be tested for COVID, as they try not to be identified as a hospital with a high number of infections. My phone feels hot, crackling with the energy of a thousand frustrated voices.

Alongside that, I'm seeing footage of pubs and clubs showing groups of people "getting their last drinks in" – crowds everywhere, even as the virus is breaking hard across London. It's as if the hospitals are at the front of the train, already nose-diving off a cliff, while some of the general public are in the drinks carriage at the back, totally unaware of the fate that befalls them.

I try to turn this feeling of helplessness and frustration at the powers that be into something constructive, to the charity, drafting and redrafting the steps to launch it as I get ready for work. I leave Dilsan with the kids around the kitchen table, drawing diagrams and plans. She looks beautiful and focused. We can all use the distraction, I suppose.

Thinking of Beck, alone in her flat now, I call her on the way to the station.

"Beck. Come and stay at ours. We are going to get locked down soon."

"I know, I've just seen an army truck going past the flat."

"Come now – it could be announced tonight. The spin studio will close soon anyway."

"Yeah, I know. Just a little longer here. I've got to tidy up."

That's so typical of Beck. She'd sweep the floors during a hurricane.

"No, Beck, come now. We don't know when we'll be allowed to travel next afterwards."

"Okay, okay. I'll come today. You finally get what you want."

"To get you to live in our attic, and to stop working at the spin studio and focus on your music?"

"Yes."

"And all it took was a global pandemic."

Beck laughs, and rings off. In the midst of the chaos it's a cheering thought, to know that Dilsan and Beck will be together, especially as they get on so well. I'll know that Beck is safe and looked after, the kids can see their Aunty "Buckie", as Ayla is wont to call her, and I can stop worrying about her being alone in the midst of the pandemic.

* * *

The tube is very quiet, and I am *en route* to the nuclear medicine department* of our hospital, as part of our training to interpret and understand how we take pictures of the heart. Even though there is a plan to move into intensive care and the rota is changing on a daily basis, these activities are the last vestiges of normality clinging on before the deluge. We can scan the heart in nearly 10 different ways, and one involves injecting radioactive dye, which tracks the blood supply through the heart muscle at rest and under stress, to give us an idea of whether a blockage in an artery might be impeding blood flow.

When I finally find my way down to the radiology department, I'm a little late. I'm expecting to see a line of waiting patients, but the waiting area is empty. I wander inside and the place literally feels like a bunker – we're under street level, the

---

* A specialized area of radiology that uses small amounts of radioactive substances to examine the physiological processes of diseases

doors are reinforced to protect from the radioactive dyes used in the scanner, and for some inexplicable reason a stockpile of bottled water and boxes of Mini Cheddars has been stacked against a wall in the reporting area. I find one other doctor, hanging around sheepishly like me. I introduce myself:

"Hi. I'm Dom, one of the cardiology registrars."

"Khalil, I'm a radiologist."

Khalil has been seconded to a special training placement from another London hospital. With time to kill, we get to chatting, inevitably about coronavirus. I'm intrigued to know in detail what other hospitals are doing.

"There are quite a few cases at our hospital now," Khalil tells me.

"How do you know?"

"Oh, the Trust email us every day, exactly how many."

I make a mental note of that as an excellent idea.

"I heard you guys have several consultants here on ITU?" Khalil asks.

I laugh, about to ask Khalil the exact same question. The same rumour seems to be flying around in ever-recycled forms, so easy to get caught up in.

"I heard that was *your* hospital. Did you hear about Northwick Park?"

"Yeah, they sound pretty busy."

"It seems wild that we are both here, learning to do a scan we probably won't be doing for months anyway."

Khalil shrugs.

"It's an oil tanker. It'll take a while to turn." He's got a point there.

The consultant arrives shortly after, a big bear of a man called Dr D'Souza, not someone I've worked with before but who I know well from various courses in the past.

"Dom – did they stick you down here?" he asks.

"That's right. Well, you seem to have the only fully stocked bunker for the apocalypse," I say, nodding to the stacks of food in the corner.

"Ah, that was Petre. Christmas party gone wrong." Dr D'Souza laughs at that. He doesn't seem at all perturbed by the world. "Now, shall we have a coffee? No patients till 11, it looks like."

We make a coffee, and wait for the patients to turn up. In the meantime, I spend some time drawing up some more charity bits. Dilsan pings me some ideas for taglines and some possible supporters.

"Did you see this?" she texts. She sends me a picture of Richard Horton, the editor of *The Lancet*, calling for help for NHS workers.

"Definitely someone we should approach," I reply.

"Yup. Also, I assume you've seen this?" She pings me a letter from NHS England. I haven't read it, actually, and I share it with the radiology team while we're sipping coffee. It's instructional advice for all clinicians, conveying the need to free up beds, especially in critical care; to expect "large numbers" of COVID-19 patients needing respiratory support; and to support staff. The last line of the letter, "Remove routine burdens so as to facilitate the above", catches my eye. Funds have been promised, and routine bureaucracy has been postponed. Long may it continue, I think to myself.

Another message lands in my phone, from my sister.

"Army on the streets in Clapham. What do you think is going on?"

A photo of the backs of two dozen olive-clad soldiers marching in pairs down Clapham High Street accompanies it. I show my phone to Dr D'Souza, who is taken aback by that.

"Closing the city?" he remarks.

I nod. It seems sensible given the scale of the outbreak already, but it may be too late. At least it will send the right message to those gallivanting in pubs every night.

I text Beck back.

"Have you left yet?!"

"Just sorting some bits. On my way!"

*　*　*

We finish at lunchtime. I've got admin time scheduled for the afternoon, and I say my goodbyes to Khalil and Dr D'Souza and start heading home, nearly walking headlong into Dilsan's maternal aunt and uncle, Narin and Hussain. Hussain had a major cardiac operation only very recently, and is coming for a follow-up scan. They are wearing gloves and masks and carrying hand sanitizer, incidentally lemon-flavoured, which is a very Turkish thing and a pleasant homely reminder when they offer to splash some on me. It's such an odd coincidence, and it feels even stranger to social distance with family, but I'm very conscious to stay well apart. They've come such a long way, I'm glad they at least took precautions getting here. We chat for a while, but they are already late for their appointment, so I promise to speak to them later. There must be so many patients in the same boat, battling through the pandemic to get to their routine appointments. How will we cope with the usual work, with so much more work to do? I know the answer, deep down. We won't.

I call Dilsan on the way home. We are running low on essentials and, busy with looking after the kids, she hasn't been able to get to the shops. Frustratingly and suddenly, Beck cancels her plan to move to ours at the last minute, still tied up "sorting a few more bits". I worry that she will leave it too late. Dilsan is very relieved to hear I'm coming home.

"Can you get here quickly? Bring food," she asks.

On the way home, I nip into the local Turkish supermarket; it's packed. There are long queuing crowds I've never seen in here before, and it's clear from their bewildered and manic searching of the aisles that many have never been in here before either. Despite being something of a secret outlet for many of the local residents, the shelves are nearly bare. I manage to scrape some unfamiliarly branded pasta, imported flour and a lot of canned beans. There are a few vegetables left and, funnily enough, there's lots of our favourite food left, like the Turkish beef sausage sucuk. Grateful that something has survived the purge, I queue and wait, crammed in a 30-person-long line, posting a few tweets about social distancing without irony. It feels like we are just making the pandemic worse, at least in London – with panic-buying crowds and rebellious pub-goers. There's a disconnect between what we are seeing with our own eyes in hospitals and what the wider public are seeing. This can't last much longer, I hope, as I pay and head home.

* * *

Once I'm home again, Dilsan and I continue fleshing out the charity idea. She's got the whiteboard pens out again, and I can see the difference as our focus shifts from the rumours flying around on our phones to something tangible and doable in front of us. We need a lot of parts immediately: a launch video, a website, a fundraising site, a mission statement. We'll need to pull in all sorts of favours to get this going right away. Like trying to do anything fast, I reach out to those closest to me, texting the message "I need a favour, mate. How do you want to help with coronagate?" to three of my best friends from school: Jack Chute, Jack Terry and Tom Parker. They all agree to drop what they're doing. Jack Chute especially jumps in with both feet, messaging back straight away.

"What's the plan?" he asks.

It's an incredibly soul-feeding activity, to ask for something and for the answer to be an unequivocal, emphatic YES.

"Trying to set up a charity/platform to support NHS staff. Might need a promo video."

"Sounds bangin'. Lemme know how I can help."

"So, if you're up for it we operate a trust policy. I trust you to come up with whatever you think is good. I just need it ASAP."

Jack is now a professional filmmaker, but funnily enough, we started out together messing around with a handheld camera and a bootlegged copy of Adobe Premiere, cutting together videos and adding effects to give us superpowers or recreate video games. I split my A-levels in half, Biology and Chemistry to cover the medicine, but also English Literature and Media Studies, simply because I enjoyed them so much. Jack and I were quite competitive at the time, although even then he blew everyone else away. Fifteen years later, Jack's a super-pro, and here he is, dropping everything to help.

It takes Jack 15 minutes to get back to me, messaging "Okay, so here's what we do."

He starts explaining how we can very rapidly cut a script featuring lots of colleagues, outlining something straightforward, a simple expression of what we want to do. In the next hour, we've drafted a script and sent out instructions. It's another school friend, Ed Terry, whose branding company designs our logo and corrects the acronym: Healthcare Extraordinary Response Organisation, *Education* and Support (HEROES). Tom agrees to build the first iteration of the website. We are already getting there.

"It's coming together," Dilsan says. "Let's call Nej?"

When we speak to Nej that evening, he's immediately stoked, but, ever the executive, very practical.

"Okay, I'm in," he says, as we are huddled around the speaker-phone going through the slides. "We'll need a clear plan, and a launch date."

"I want to launch it on Friday."

"Wow, okay, that's punchy. Can we do that?"

"Jack is cutting a video for us, we have the fundraising website going, and Barky [Tom's affectionate nickname] is building a website for us. We can do this."

"Okay. Let's do it. Let's have a call again tomorrow night to see where we are."

It's late, and Dilsan and I both feel like we've run a marathon. I ping a brief about the charity to Beck.

"This is your new job," I write underneath it.

"Okay, boss," she answers, straight away.

"Thank you for interviewing. You have been successful. Congratulations."

"Looks great. What do you need?"

Beck is in too. The team is coming together.

* * *

Dilsan calls over from the living room.

"Do you know Roshana Mehdian? She's started a childcare co-op for NHS workers."

"Rosh and I worked together on the junior doctors' strikes* a few years ago – I think I still have her number." I message her that evening before bed, asking if she wants to get involved in the charity.

"How are Nesli and Ehsan doing?" I ask.

"Shall we give them a call?"

"It's a bit late."

"Let's try them," Dilsan says, dialling their number. Nes picks up after one ring.

"We were just messaging you guys!" Nes pipes up on the speakerphone.

We laugh. It feels good. Nesli and Ehsan ask about the government measures announced on Monday (16 March, when Boris announced that schools would close for all children except those of key workers).

"The announcement was good, right?" Ehsan says.

"Not enough, I reckon. But things are changing," I say.

---

* The long-running dispute between 2015 and 2016 over the government's proposed imposition of a new contract for junior doctors

"Yeah, did you see this?" Ehsan pings me a news story. "ISIS have recommended their terrorists don't travel."

"Bloody hell! ISIS are being stricter about travel in coronavirus than we are," I say.

It's stupid, and hilarious. Exhausted, we ring off. To be finally doing something positive is exciting, but more than that, it's calming.

• • •

The following morning, the situation is worsening quickly across London. My doctors' groups are a mix, ranging from the incredibly scared to the blasé, as well as those burying their heads and just trying to keep the service going. A few are trying to be proactive, trying to get the message across to those who still don't get the severity of the situation. The scientific data suggests that while younger patients are the least likely to be seriously unwell, they are the most likely to be asymptomatic spreaders. Those newsreel clips of pubs full of young people feel like a knife being twisted in. The government needs to step in.

Meanwhile, there is some good news filtering through by email and WhatsApp – Jack has sent through an early version of the launch video and it's incredibly moving. We've even got Ralf Little from *The Royle Family*-fame to make a cameo. Also, Ed has put together some logos for the charity, and it's the first time we see the colours and the design. Dilsan is really pleased and okays all the design work. Beck sends us a picture of her packed bags, and a message that says "cominnggg!" Despite everything else that's going on, I leave the house feeling determined, with Dilsan absorbed in the charity work. We are laying the track as we go, but at least there's a destination to get to.

As the week winds to a close, it seems that more and more commuters have disappeared from the daily grind. The tube is deserted, and as I come out of the station, the streets are sparsely populated. Overnight, I was sent a long list of discounts for NHS workers; coffee shops are offering 50 per cent off drinks and free food, and restaurants are heavily discounted. I take up the offer in the local Pret, as the other coffee shops in the street have closed already. All the tables and chairs have been removed, and two lonely staff are manning the till in the otherwise deserted shop. I get a coffee and free breakfast for under £1. I feel oddly self-conscious pulling out my ID – in this deeply uncertain time, I wonder if I will be more of a pariah than a welcome customer. I can't read much from the baristas – they both just look deflated and a little scared.

I'm due in the echo department again this morning, but there are now nearly no patients. I sit in the back office and chat to Jack the echo tech, while I try to sort out my logbook. And then I start working on HEROES again, as we launch tomorrow. As I'm looking up the paperwork to apply to become a charity, one of the senior registrars comes in, Nicole. Nicole came to the UK from Singapore to go to medical school, and her whole family are still there. Growing up during SARS, she and her family know first-hand about pandemics. We get to chatting about how the UK compares.

"Are you joking?" she starts. "In Singapore, everyone wears a mask, and in hospitals, they all wear full personal protective equipment: suit, mask and eyewear, for every suspected patient. They haven't had a single hospital-acquired staff infection."

"Why aren't we doing that here?" I ask.

"This is just standard stuff in Singapore, I suppose – they are used to it, especially after SARS. And prepared. We are neither, here."

"What do your family think about us?"

"They couldn't believe the guidance here – they are trying to send us thousands of masks, but there's some more imported cases over there so it might be difficult."

"Oh. Well, let me know about the masks." I tell her about the charity. "Maybe we can get some in on a bigger scale?"

"Will do, Dom. Good luck."

"You too, Nic."

Nicole disappears to her actual job, and I finish up with my logbook.

I spend the afternoon trying to help the more junior doctors get their fit-testing and test access sorted for the weekend, sending WhatsApps and emails. Everyone has the same sense of impending doom, but, being a referral hospital, only taking patients from other hospitals and without a direct A&E ourselves, we are sitting in the eye of the storm, waiting our turn. We don't have long to wait.

• • •

On the way home, like dominoes, a series of messages arrives, bowing to the inevitable. Four friends, all doctors, cancel their weddings, only a few weeks away, along with the stag do I was particularly looking forward to, even if I had already resigned myself to the fact it was unlikely to go ahead weeks ago. We arrange a drink on Zoom instead, and set a date for next week. Hannah, the bride-to-be and an infectious disease registrar, puts it most succinctly when she writes in her email: "Corona has taken a big shit on 2020."

I get home in the middle of the afternoon and Ayla and Dilsan are sitting on the couch, painting their toenails. There's no sign of Beck yet.

"What happened to Beck?" I ask.

Dilsan shrugs. "I'll text her."

In the meantime, Ayla decides that I need painted toenails as well, and very carefully and luridly paints the toenails of my left foot in an eclectic mix of peach, bright yellow, maroon and an aquamarine that continues past the nail bed. "Pandemic toes", I call it. It's a horrible sight, but Ayla is very pleased. I like the idea – it's a little piece of home to take to work, a talisman to protect me and a token to remind me.

Beck texts Dilsan back. She says she's been doing some work on the charity already, linking in to her new job to support transaction fee-less donation, with a company called BANKED. She's spoken to Brad and Les (the CEO and his wife) and they love the idea. Even now, apparently with the Army on the streets, I feel like Beck is still stalling. She's as stubborn as I am, but I think she's coming round.

Jack checks in and attaches the final edit of the launch video – it's hauntingly beautiful. The website is now up and running, too. Roshana messages back – she's keen to be involved in the charity and, already working on her childcare co-op, has set up a legal team and is far more advanced in that regard than us. I ask her if she wants to be a trustee, and she accepts. Everything is ready now, as we plan to launch the video and GoFundMe on Twitter the next day. At least that's the plan. We catch up with Nej again late that night and work out a strategy for how we should present ourselves.

"The best thing for NHS workers is for us to be supportive and to work with the government," he says.

I agree. "Yes, the ship is turning now anyway, and we are trying to all work together. And we want to be able to help with PPE without picking a fight."

"Exactly. It's a positive message and people will want to get behind that, especially right now. There will be time for the inquiries later."

I can't sleep again that night, with too much activity on my phone. Just after midnight on Friday 20 March, I release the launch video on Twitter. We are live now, and very much committed.

By 4 a.m., we've raised £1,000. By 9.30 a.m., it's at £5,000.

As I head back into work again, the trains are deserted – Friday is normally quiet anyway, but my messages and groups are so active, it feels noisy. Rosh, Beck, Dilsan, Nej and I start a WhatsApp group to introduce everyone and to start coordinating. Beck promises to finally come to ours today. Everyone is working full-steam in 17 different directions.

"My head hurts. (Cos of this not coronavirus)," Rosh messages with a smile emoticon.

"It feels like we started a fire," Dilsan replies.

"Yup! No turning back now!" Beck adds. "So many people want to help. £10k already!"

My DMs are flooded with offers of help; professional therapists from Harley Therapy want to give 600 free hours a week to

NHS workers. I pencil a phone call in for lunchtime. Another group of medical students called NHS Supporters are setting up a childcare portal, and Rosh offers to link in with them. NHS Charities Together reaches out to us. They are launching their own campaign that evening and I'm really keen to cooperate – I certainly don't want to compete – but equally a large and fractured charity model like theirs won't be able to do what we want to do, specifically organize the supply of PPE and deliver it directly to NHS workers. We set up a call for later in the afternoon. Meanwhile, a Cambridge University final-year medical student called Ravi Solanki messages me; Ravi is already heavily embedded in the start-up tech scene in the UK, and well underway with his own website called stopthespread. info to educate and share COVID information. He has a team of 30 volunteers based around the world and offers to help us.

The streets are empty when I come out of the station. It's eerie. It feels like the opening scenes in *28 Days Later*, walking out to find a deserted London, stripped of life. The coffee shops are closed. The hospital is starting to shift and reorganize, and the front door is now closed, redirecting people around the side through a handwashing station. The echo department is a ghost town as well – very few patients are on the list for the morning. We are wearing gloves and visors but no masks as yet, and each patient needs to be clear of fever and symptoms before we chivvy them into the examination room. Sitting in a dark room, staring at the grey-white pictures of a beating heart muscle, trying to optimize depth, gain, sector width and a dozen other controls, takes my full concentration. It's even meditative, to have some time forced away from my phone and the fire we've started elsewhere. For Dilsan, Beck, Nej and Rosh, the fire is still burning. I get the sense it'll be like this a lot going forward, especially as I join the intensive care rota next week – disappearing to work and leaving the others to deal with running the charity. There isn't much media interest yet – a charity that hasn't raised any substantial money or really done anything so far is just an idea with a website, I suppose. It'll come, I hope. We hit £20,000 in donations by lunchtime.

Meanwhile, the wave continues to crash. A local ICU has already had to triple capacity, and the news about Northwick Park Hospital running out of ICU beds is being reported in mainstream media, quoting a "senior director" reflecting that "this is f**king petrifying" – a sentiment that so many of us are feeling. There's real debate about the value of being "reassuring" at this point, when so many Londoners clearly don't need to be "reassured" as much as presented with the stark truth of what's actually going on in hospitals as soon as possible. The sheer velocity of the situation is unimaginable, and every day feels newly horrifying. Nine days ago, I'd tweeted that we were 10 days away from "hospital meltdown". I'm sad to realize that it came even sooner. I message this to Dilsan.

"It's only been nine days."

"I know. We are majorly in trouble here," she texts back.

"It's okay, we are doing what we can," I reply.

"Beck is finally here at least. So much better with another pair of hands."

I'm hugely relieved. At least Beck has finally landed at ours and we can begin the bunkering down that so many families are contemplating.

For Nesli and Ehsan, they have had the confirmation that their schools will be closing, and are trying to work out how they can shield all together. They're facing a long stretch where the only realistic way to protect Ehsan and stay together is to lock themselves away, essentially cocooning the whole family for months on end, in a small house and with two kids under five. A "hard" lockdown is inevitable, but at least for me the hours at home will be filled, even stuffed, with the charity, and I can still legitimately go outside, to go to work. I worry how tolerable it'll be for everyone. Though with nearly 4,000 cases now reported, and with 250 people already having lost their lives, if we don't lock down properly soon, it'll be catastrophic.

Anaesthetic consultant Michelle Dawson messages me when I'm halfway home. It turns out local hospitals are being told they can't purchase extra PPE for themselves, but she's decided to keep trying to prod NHS procurement to allow it. In addition to this problem, the ICU in her hospital was blocked from buying specialized hoods with visors (equipment usually worn by welders) by another department within the hospital, infection control.

"Trusts are worried they will be sued if they go outside the supply chain. Need to be more nimble here. What can we do?"

"Let me see what I can find out," I reply, sending a few messages to some of the legal supporters that have reached out to help us.

It's disheartening to immediately run into bureaucratic and political barriers – there's a disconnected intransigence to the concept of adaptation, a stymying "business as usual" attitude that infuriates.

By the time I get home, Beck is well settled ("haunting the attic", as she puts it) and working hard on the charity. Our cupboards are once again adorned with writing and the weather outside is cuttingly cold, but the house is filled with the warm smell of chicken curry. Not working for once this weekend, due to the stopping of cross-site safari shifts, I have a chance to stop and catch up. I speak to Ravi on the phone – he's seen our campaign, and wants to repurpose his entire team over the weekend to create a bespoke website for us. By Monday. It's a gargantuan effort. I'm really touched by his commitment and sincerity. I invite him to join the board.

We have our first board meeting that evening, huddled in the kitchen on Zoom, myself, Nej, Dilsan, Beck, Rosh, Ravi, Michelle, Ed and Jack. It's only day one but feels like we have been going for months. There's an uplifting, hopeful energy, and also wine. It's really nice to speak to other real, non-medical people again. We realize we've missed the government's daily briefing for the first time in a long time; it somehow seems less important. We know where we are going now and there's a very long way to get there.

. . .

Nej calls us in the morning – he has a family connection to Joe Cole, ex-England footballer and television pundit. After a kitchen conversation about the charity, Joe and his wife Carly both want to help, to join as our founding ambassadors. Over the weekend we scramble to get the website ready, to chase up our PPE leads, to start a food service, to link in childcare services. It's a crazy, creative, consuming effort. Joe and his people arrange Friday morning (27 March) slots on "Good Morning Britain" and "BBC Breakfast".

My friend Jack Chute calls me on the Saturday afternoon – he has a connection with the same projectionists that worked on the Led By Donkeys campaign,* and they want to get involved with the charity as well. We draw up some plans that day, to broadcast a thousand-foot launch video for our charity onto a national monument or building. We talk about locations and one strikes me as ludicrous, but it becomes more and more appropriate as I think about it: the White Cliffs of Dover. The association with the war, that symbol of British togetherness in the face of adversity: it's the right location. We agree to put together another video overnight – Jack is pulling all-nighters to get the edits and the momentum going. And so, their team plots to get a video up on Sunday night, planning to carefully trek down to the shore with tens of thousands of pounds of equipment, to shoot a football-pitch-size picture of our charity. When we film our contribution, Zach keeps wanting to be picked up, so he ends up in the video, being carried around, to get our submission in on time.

The news from the outside world, which feels ever more remote, is bleak. There are reports of NHS workers being mugged for their IDs in central London, presumably fuelled by the rumours that a hard lockdown is coming and an NHS ID pass will be the only means of travel. I find it physically sickening. It feels like a kick in the teeth, when we are already having

---

* The political campaign group, formed in December 2018, that were responsible for projecting satirical messages on the Houses of Parliament that were seen by millions. The name comes from the expression "lions led by donkeys" from the First World War, used to describe the brave infantrymen and the clueless generals sending them to their deaths

to deal with so much. Trusts are advising caution and partnering up for walks to and from tube stations, particularly at night.

As if the situation couldn't get any worse, we hear about the first seemingly confirmed colleague of ours who is critically unwell with COVID-19. An announcement from the British Laryngological Association reports that at least two ear, nose and throat (ENT) surgeons are critically unwell. ENT doctors seem to be particularly at risk, given their close proximity to the highest-risk areas of infection – the mouth and nose mucosa. The news drops into our timelines like a stone. A colleague writes a comment underneath it – "Stay safe, we aren't of use to anyone if we are dead" – that makes me think. I suppose we all have to adjust our normal attitudes at work. Someone posts underneath a link to a thread on Twitter titled "There is no emergency in a pandemic", describing this idea of protecting oneself first before rushing to an unwell patient. We are faced with a potentially overwhelming patient burden, and healthcare workers become force multipliers of good in that situation – their continued good health ensures the good health of tens if not hundreds of patients. If a healthcare worker, particularly one with vital expertise such as intensive care, becomes ill, they go from providing that healthcare resource to using resources themselves. They also leave behind hard-to-fill gaps, stretching already stretched colleagues, which leads to mistakes, and potentially more unwell colleagues. There is no emergency in a pandemic.

Even cardiac arrest, the most critical emergency, is dangerous to healthcare workers in an infected or suspected patient, due to the aerosols generated with each compression of the chest, and members of the team need to don protective equipment before starting life-saving CPR (cardiopulmonary resuscitation). Hesitating in this situation feels inherently wrong, and the idea of stopping to put on masks, gloves and gowns is very difficult to swallow. But we will all have to adjust to what is likely to be months if not years of pandemic care. It's simply the new normal.

The world is changing.

Dilsan finds me staring at my phone.

"C'mon, we need to have this call with Nej's contact at the meat company," she reminds me.

We are trying to arrange for cost-price food drops for NHS staff to counter the difficulty of getting to the shops. Sainsbury's have just announced a specific time for NHS workers, but have combined it with the hour for elderly workers, which strikes us all as a very bad idea, mixing the most exposed with the most vulnerable.

"We should be getting the supermarkets to prioritize online shopping for healthcare workers," I say.

"Well, let's start here and work from there?" Dilsan replies.

It just seems like everything we try to do is on such a small scale compared to the mountain of need. We have 1.5 million healthcare workers, needing something like a billion sets of PPE a month and millions of meals a day. Thousands of these workers have been infected already and at least one has already passed away, and there's a mounting wave of infection still to hit. Dilsan senses my frustration.

"We do what we can – we won't be able to do everything."

We share a smile. It was me telling her the same yesterday, and she's right, of course. And it helps to even do the smallest thing. We arrange food boxes for several NHS workers to go out that week, as a trial. It's such a small thing, but it's deeply satisfying to try to help.

We have another call that night. Already the team is twice the size it was yesterday. Ravi's team has drafted the bespoke website, in just over a day. The pace is truly blistering, and it looks fantastic. Michelle has another lead who might be able to supply 30 million masks a month and is working on getting through to NHS procurement. Joe and Carly Cole are our ambassadors, and Piers Morgan is going to mention the charity the next day on "Good Morning Britain". The fire is burning bigger and brighter. It feels a lot like trying to build a bicycle that you are already cycling down a very steep hill, realizing you need pedals and brakes as you reach for them, and just as quickly those parts are there, and you are then going even faster, gathering momentum.

• • •

I wake up in the morning, early, with the sun streaming in. The days are getting longer and the morning reaches into our room with a bright, yellow-orange glow. I check my phone – it's just past 6 a.m. Mercifully, there's no sign of the kids yet, and Dilsan is sleeping quietly next to me. I steal downstairs, opening the door carefully to avoid pushing into Max, our cat, who is always waiting too close to be fed. Piers Morgan said he'd mention the charity this morning, so I set the TV up on a low volume, trying to puzzle through the live subtitles what they are talking about. The whole downstairs is bathed in that same light; it's a stunning day, and so quiet for a Monday morning – there's no traffic, the schools are closed so there's no school run, no one even walking their dog. Just the bird-song to listen to.

Much as I think I've got up early, the website team have worked all night to get the website live, and it sits there in a beautiful blue and white motif. The Dover team have pulled an all-nighter as well, and Jack has sent me some snaps of the shoot, the White Cliffs imposing with our logo projected widely across it. Nej has been commenting on our charity WhatsApp operations group, already awake at 5 a.m. I wonder at his energy and drive, thinking we are very lucky to have him. In my reverie of looking at my phone, I worry I've missed any mention of us on the TV. It doesn't matter – despite the overwhelmingly dire situation, in the quiet, wrapped in a blanket, with a mug of tea, everything seems manageable. I had booked annual leave this week, although it's been inter-rupted by two days of intensive care training bolted on at the last minute, starting tomorrow. The thought gives my Zen mood a wobble.

Dilsan comes down with Zach. He wriggles to get to me with a big smile on his face when they appear.

"Good morning," Dilsan says sleepily. She sees "Good Morning Britain" in the background, a show we never watch. "Anything about the charity?" she asks.

"I'm not sure. Think I missed it if there was. Website is up – have a look," I say.

Dilsan flicks through her phone.

"Wow. They did this in two days?"

"It's amazing, isn't it? They've been up all night. They all have. They just want to help."

"Did you see this, by the way?" Dilsan passes me her phone. "I posted in my mum's group about the charity, asking if anyone had any contacts to help with getting the 30 million masks from China."

"And?"

"I've got a private message back – an email. It looks like it's from the Cabinet Office."

A new team has been assembled there, looking at extra-NHS supply line procurement. I email them immediately, and within minutes a reply comes back, with a mobile number.

I ring it straight away – it's only just past 7 a.m. It rings through to a civil servant, running a new team to source PPE outside of the traditional supply lines. It seems someone in government is getting it. The hairs on the back of my neck stand up to hear how switched-on and keen she is to connect with Michelle, and to get these large volumes of masks from China – properly fit-tested masks which could prevent any more of my colleagues from catching the virus, as well as protecting hospices and GPs. We chat briefly about other offers to produce masks – from industry or from donors. We agree to work together; we will offer the government first refusal to any suppliers that come through us offering to manufacture masks in very large quantities. We can arrange to distribute smaller quantities ourselves, as well. I connect Michelle and her contact. I tell Dilsan, my voice breaking a bit when I mention the details – we feel like we've made a real contribution here, even just to join the dots like this.

Shortly after Ayla is up, the WhatsApp groups start firing off, and it's pandemonium again. Beck has been leveraging her never-ending list of PR/tech/legal contacts – she's been working herself to the bone on this like everyone else. It's deeply soul-feeding work, but there's also a lot of pressure involved to deliver, to get masks out to the frontline as soon as possible. It's chaotic – trying to manage a team that is doubling faster than the virus, every day, with different roles and responsibilities and lots of personalities. Inevitably we end up bumping into each other, confusing jobs, organizing two separate PR teams, missing emails. It isn't at all easy.

Michelle messages me about the person in the government, who has connected directly to her own contact. I cross all my fingers and toes that this will go somewhere. She also messages me about another initiative, called Contractors Appeal, and wonders if we should connect. They are a group of contractors in the building industry, trying to source and deliver PPE to NHS workers. Michelle explains a bit about PPE used outside of hospitals, and how an FFP mask in the hospital was exactly the same as an FFP mask on a construction site – the numbering system (FFP1, FFP2 and FFP3) was just a measure of the particulate size that was filtered, whether that was protecting from drops of virus or clouds of dust. I email Paul Ford from Contractors Appeal that morning, and he comes back to me, asking to have a chat at 10.30 a.m.

Sitting in my kitchen, making Zoom calls, with bedlam in the background, already feels like a "new normal". As Paul pops into the screen for the first time, sitting in his kitchen, conservatory in the background, it feels like we are all in the same world now. Paul Ford has a generous warmth and humility that belies his incredibly accomplished background; he's the Chairman of the De Group, a company with a value of £120 million. He was also one of the first civilians to visit Grenfell. Paul is the living embodiment of the pragmatic "can-do" attitude that we all need in the midst of an emergency. We discuss how we can work together, possibly with another group called Med Supply Drive. I suggest we set up a regular meeting with all the PPE groups and coordinate requests and resources. We aim to set up a call later in the week.

That's when I decide to check the charity's GoFundMe page and see we've raised nearly £75,000. Several large donations are starting to give it real momentum. We could make such a difference here.

Michelle messages me – she's sceptical that industry can supply the volumes we will need, but it gets me to wondering what else we could be doing. Maybe we could make things? Ehsan brought a 3D printer home a few months ago, and I've been desperate to play with it. The idea of a future technology like this, capable of printing anything in an emergency, seems wacky and wonderful. I've seen some US companies already making 3D-printed respirators and snorkel mask conduits to create DIY masks. I wonder if anyone is doing the same in the UK. I tweet asking for some help.

More good news comes during the day: GoFundMe are donating £5,000 to us to cover their platform costs, which they can't waive, and the childcare co-op has already matched 200 families to childcare. Boris Johnson is due on at 8.30 p.m., so we have our now-regular board meeting snappily and sit down to watch the pre-recorded message. It's an expected announcement, but hearing the emphatic "you now must stay at home" feels like a huge relief, enforcing the lockdown and closing schools, shops, and places of worship. Stay at home if you can.

Dilsan is cuddled up next to me on the couch.

"Is it enough?"

"It's too late. But no more to do now."

I really hope it's enough; it feels like it took a lifetime coming down the line.

"Just have to get on with it now, I guess."

I start ICU training in the morning. We are both aware of it. We watch the television a little more in silence.

CHAPTER 7

Critical

The morning isn't the ghost town I expect to see – when I change at Finsbury Park, the station is packed three–four deep, mostly young men, many of whom, from the look of the equipment they're carrying, are manual workers. Without any way to work from home, what was expected, though? I can't understand why the train is still so packed – surely some commuters must've stayed home after last night's announcement. My friends message me with much the same news, mentioning that the Central line is packed and remarking that the lockdown is hard to enforce. It's a bright, warm morning, but the crowds are ominous. I later find out that the tube has been running fewer trains, sardining more people into smaller spaces; it seems so short-sighted. By the time I exit the station I'm deeply unsettled. The coffee shops are closed and my morning ritual is in tatters. This is not a good start to the day. I wander into the hospital in a grey mood, get changed into the familiar scrubs, and then take the lift upstairs, to intensive care.

● ● ●

I've worked in intensive care before, four dark months over a winter rotation several years ago, and much of the skills and training is similar to what we already do in cardiology: putting lines into arteries and veins, and managing low blood pressures and failing hearts with drugs to make the heart pump better. As I nervously look for the handover room, seek out unfamiliar faces and sit awkwardly in a new room waiting for a shift I feel totally unprepared for, it feels like my first ever day as a doctor all over again. That memory blossoms vividly in my mind, though it feels like two lifetimes ago.

When we first started as doctors, we spent days "shadowing" – following the "real" docs around, who were only a year ahead of us, but what a difference a year made. During that first shadow-week, we were just ghosts waiting for the moment that we would be made real. That moment came too soon, though. On the penultimate day of crossover, when we were just about to enter the hospital for the first time as fully-fledged doctors, the doctors at the end of their first years were doing their rounds like a victory lap, saying their goodbyes, confidently swaggering from patient to patient and ward to ward with a practised ease gained from months of graft. The same months that we had ahead of us, and felt totally unready for. We were performing rounds in the surgical department, attending to patients awaiting or recovering from surgeries to their stomach, bowels or vessels. That afternoon, I had my training wheels removed and swerved unsteadily around the place, trying to do the jobs like taking bloods and placing lines for medicines (cannulas) that would be my responsibility tomorrow. Somewhere down the ward, the real deal doctor I was following, Robert, was attending to another patient. While I scuttled past, the senior sister on the ward, Siobhan, grabbed my arm and directed me to a young woman called Florence who'd just returned from the operating theatre. She'd come in for a simple procedure to have an abscess drained, but it had required a general anaesthetic.

"Her oxygen is a little low, let's go see her?"

In medical school we were taught to deal with emergencies in a very structured, focused way. We learnt and chanted mantras to avert catastrophe: Look. Listen. Feel. Treat. Repeat. DR ABCDE.* These incantations got trotted out as the gears in our heads ground away, and by the time we came to final exams, the machine in our heads was primed. You fed the instructions in and out came the response. Going to assess Florence was such a simple task, one that I'd practised and even been examined on a hundred times before, and yet, when Siobhan wheeled me around to see her, I just froze. I fed the scenario to those same gears in my head and they stalled, whirred, and then pinged into the darkness. I reached for instructions and found nothing. All I could do was stare at her as she lay slumped in her bed, with the little oxygen probe next to her flashing gently "89%". I could almost feel Siobhan's mental prod in my back.

"Oxygen?" I suggested weakly. We put a mask on Florence's face, her wispy blonde hair matted to her forehead. And then I had nothing. I just stared at her, willed her to breathe. The gaps between those breaths were too long, chasms I could feel my whole medical career up to that moment falling into.

---

* **D**anger, **R**esponse, **A**irway, **B**reathing, **C**PR, **D**isability, **E**verything else

Thankfully, Siobhan nipped over to fetch Robert, who confidently strode past, examined Florence's chest and flashed a pen torch into each eye. She groaned and turned to the other side of the bed.

"Siobhan, can I have some naloxone, please?"

Siobhan was ready behind with a pre-drawn syringe and an expression that only a senior nurse of 10 years-plus experience can truly give.

Robert fiddled with her IV line, and within a minute, Florence was leaning forward, bright-eyed.

Florence yawned loudly. "Can I go home now?" she asked.

Robert made a quick plan.

"No more morphine, supportive care for now, keep the monitor on and we'll review in 30 minutes or so."

Siobhan gave me a level look as she walked away.

Rob gave me a different, knowing one. "Pub?" he asked.

Back in the present, eight years later, I get that same paralyzing flutter in my chest as we sit waiting for our briefing, outside intensive care. There's a whole mix of doctors here from outside the intensive care: not just cardiology registrars, but lung doctors, cancer doctors, kidney doctors, surgeons. And not just junior doctors either – several consultants are sitting here too, willing to re-train to do what they can to help with the pandemic. Some of the consultants aren't too far from retirement, in a far higher-risk group than me. I can't help but admire their courage, given that I was anxious to come to ICU, and I'm 32 in a low-risk group. And yet here they are, as ready to learn a new skill set and help as everyone else. Currently our hospital is receiving patients from other places – we are the spill-over – and there's only a handful of COVID-19 patients on the ward at the moment.

The handover begins when the consultants walk in. They are Dr Duncan Desmond, the lead for the unit, and another boss I know from our occasional encounters in cardiac procedures or emergencies, Dr Lourdes.

"Welcome, everyone," says Dr Desmond. "Thank you, sincerely, for joining us to come and help. We'll do the handover, then we'll go round."

The night registrar starts reeling through the patients' stories. It's the same pitter-patter of numbers and phrases I've heard dozens of times before, only this time with a new opening, "COVID Positive" or "COVID Negative". There are more COVID patients than I've seen to date, and they account for about half of the ward. As cardiology registrars, we spend our days paying attention to the "C" (Circulation) in ABC, and often neglecting the "A" and "B" (Airway and Breathing), as they are catered for by other specialties. But now all of that is squarely part of the remit. The numbers tickle the rusty cogs stored somewhere dark and forgotten in my medical mind. The group of around 16 doctors – three or four of the regular doctors on the ICU and about a dozen doctors like me being cross-trained – files out into the corridor. There's a short lull, and little pools of conversation stir while we wait, with the occasional nervous laugh. We then divide like ducklings behind the consultants and follow them onto the ward.

Most people will never see the inside of an intensive care unit during their lifetime, and you should hope to never have to. The Faculty of Intensive Care defines a "Unit" as "a specially staffed and equipped, separate and self-contained area of a hospital dedicated to the management and monitoring of patients with life-threatening conditions". The "Intensive" treatment is the whole gamut of the most invasive, high-tech medical apparatus we have access to. There are machines to help patients breathe, and machines to replace the function of kidneys and even hearts. We put long tubes directly in veins and arteries to give multiple infusions of drugs and to monitor blood pressure beat to beat; we put tubes in bladders and bowels, and one directly into the windpipe, a process called "intubation", and another tube into the food pipe for feeding. We take blood multiple times a day, usually from a catheter inserted to maintain access to patients' veins. It's quite common for patients to become anaemic simply from the routine care in an intensive care unit. A single patient on maximum support may have 10 medicine infusions running simultaneously. Every patient will need to have 50 or so parameters recorded every hour, and this requires the expertise to not only maintain all of these machines and respond to each parameter, but also deliver all of the usual care that patients require; turning them to prevent problems associated with immobility such as bed sores, attending to their mouths and their bowels and administering medicines. Intensive care nurses are the most valuable and skilled resource in the department, a resource we are desperately short of in the UK.

We embark on our ward round and come to the first patient's bedside. A computer on wheels travels with us, and the junior doctor on the ward reels off the patient's history; it's a story I've heard too many times in my relatively short career. The man lying supine (facing upwards) before me is Abdul; he's just 45 and he drives a bus. He does not have COVID, though. After a shift two nights ago, he had been walking to the underground when he collapsed in the street. It sounds like it was a number of minutes before a passer-by started CPR – vital time that may have made the difference between him walking out of here and never walking again. When the ambulance arrived, they found his heart oscillating widely in a fatal rhythm known as ventricular fibrillation, and applied a defibrillator (essentially a mobile battery attached to two pads slapped to the chest), administering a shock to snap the heart back into a normal rhythm. It didn't work the first time, and took a further shock to restore the normal "lub-dub".

Stabilized, Abdul was whisked to his local heart centre, where tubes were placed in his windpipe and then into the artery in the wrist, and, as quickly as possible, further tubes were slid the length of the arm and chest to reach the arteries of the heart. There, they found the problem that had started all this: a blood clot, just four millimetres wide, blocking flow to the main artery of the heart. A wire was passed through the obstruction, a special tube called a stent was inserted and expanded, and blood flow was restored. But it may already have been too late, as too much time may have elapsed without circulation to the brain. Only time will tell.

A breathing tube called an endotracheal tube protrudes from between Abdul's lips, tied in place by a soft band of velcro that encircles his head. The tubing snakes out to the machine by his bedside, the Rolls-Royce of ventilators, featuring a touchscreen that resembles a desktop PC. The little numbers and figures track a dozen parameters of his breathing: the volumes going in and out, the rate and mode of the ventilator blowing oxygen into the lungs, and the amount and concentration of that oxygen. Neat coloured peaks and troughs are displayed alongside, visualizations of the numbers that allow us to see the shape and rhythm of his breathing. Above the ventilator beeps the monitor displaying his vital signs; far more things are tracked than for a usual patient in a normal hospital ward bed. There's a live electrical tracing of his heart, a monitor displaying the level of oxygen in his blood, a beat-to-beat representation of the pressures in his artery and the timing of the rise and fall of his chest. From the monitor, lines stretch back to a tube in Abdul's wrist artery to check his blood pressure, and another line is attached to an octopus of tubes in his neck. These neck tubes splay out to a dozen pumps, stacked like mini skyscrapers in towers around him, each flashing a blue dial of numbers and names, the many medicines Abdul is on to maintain his sedation, to increase his blood pressure, to control his blood sugar. On his chest are electrodes to monitor his heart and large pads to shock him again, if needed. Another tube from his penis drains his urine. He is wrapped in a temperature-controlled blanket, to keep him cool, a technique we have learnt makes brain recovery more likely. Large boots wrap around both legs to prevent blood clots. This is what "intensive" care looks like.

Dr Lourdes starts making her assessment, starting with the oversized paper chart at Abdul's bedside. Laid out like a map, the paper is crowded with a thousand numbers and figures, the product of just a single day in intensive care. Every element is recorded: his vital signs, the ventilator settings and modes, his blood acidity, oxygen and carbon dioxide levels, the sugar and the level of lactate, which is a marker of tissue damage, how much fluid goes in and out each hour, subdivided into individual inputs and outputs with a total at the bottom, how much food is coming from the stomach tube in Abdul's nose and the volume of stool removed. The volume and doses of infusions each hour and the basic observations of the position of the breathing tube are also recorded, as are the depth of sedation and the observations of brain function. As far as intensive care goes, this is just the basic chart – more advanced interventions, such as extra-corporeal membrane oxygenation (ECMO), essentially a replacement circulatory system, can also be utilized. It's a dizzying array of numbers, and my eyes strain to find the specifics when I look for them. I don't have the muscle memory yet, lack the familiar handholds I had in cardiology. I'm very much back at square one again here, and more than a little anxious for it.

We go through each parameter, examine Abdul from top to bottom thoroughly, from his eyes down to the tubes protruding from his nose, mouth and throat, to his chest, abdomen and legs. We look at the blood tests and the X-rays, the ECGs and the medicine chart. Then Dr Lourdes makes a plan, writes on the chart and sets the "targets" for the day, the parameters the ICU nurses will deploy their expertise in attaining, for example, the level of acidity or carbon dioxide in the blood or the target blood pressure. He's on the right medications, and there is little to adjust. For Abdul, the plan is to support his body and simply wait. And then we move on, recording all of that in a long entry on our electronic system. Then we go through the same motions for the next patient, and the next.

Eventually the ward round crosses over to the COVID bay,

where six patients have been cohorted into a single area. We need to put on the personal protective equipment here before entering, a process we call "donning". We've had a simulation training session, but this is the first time I've worn this stuff in real life, with the real risk of exposure. The first time we "don", it's awkward, trying to remember the steps in the right order, as we were taught. First, there are the shoe covers to prevent us from traipsing infection across the wards, and then there's a tie-back surgical hat to cover our hair. Then comes the first pair of gloves. Over that, there's a disposable gown which ties at the back and loops around the front. A second pair of gloves fits over the first. Finally, there's the mask, an FFP3 (the mask with protection against the finest, smallest particles), made of a thick cloth material, with two elastic bands, one of which fits over the nape of the neck and the other the crown of the head. Over the nose is a mouldable metal band, and we squeeze tightly to fit it flush to our face and cheeks. Lastly, there's the eye protection. It surprises me to find we only have disposable frames, attached to a flimsy acetate eye shield.

"Hold onto that one," Dr Lourdes tells me. "We don't have too many."

I gingerly pick a fetching hot-pink frame and loop it over my ears. Finally, there are the checks. One of the other doctors, an oncology doctor I've not worked with before called Helen, acts as my "buddy", checking I am properly adorned, before I do the same for her. Then we check the mask fit, by gently blowing air out and in, watching to see if the mask balloons in and out without expelling air into the face or eyes. It seems okay, but the glasses fog up nonetheless, which has me worried. We cross the threshold into the COVID area, awkwardly filing through the double doors. Before we cross, a nurse in PPE holds up a hand-written shopping list of items detailing the fluids, medicines and other supplies for the patients that they would normally get themselves but now need someone to get for them, and we relay it verbally to a 'runner'.

I'm not sure what I expected when I enter the coronavirus bay; I imagined I'd feel like I was wearing a spacesuit, claustrophobic in my astronaut-like helmet, with the sound of my breathing crashing in my ears. Or perhaps I envisaged something like the gloomy and hazy world of the Upside Down from "Stranger Things", the air thick with the spores of infection. But in reality, I find the PPE quite comfortable, familiar from wearing a mask for months prior, and it's an area I've been in dozens of times before. It's a slight relief to find that, in reality, it feels quite routine.

Our first patient is Deirdre, a retired primary school teacher in her late seventies. Dr Lourdes presents the case to us, as she knows Deirdre best.

"Deirdre was our first coronavirus patient, a non-clinical transfer from an external hospital." "Non-clinical transfer" means there was no special medical team or surgical team to transfer to, just that a bed was required from the much-busier external hospitals. "She was unwell for 10 days before presenting, intubated and ventilated in the Emergency department. History of hypertension (high blood pressure) and raised BMI."

"Raised BMI" is essentially a medically polite term for obesity. Deirdre weighs over 100 kg, which places her in a much higher-risk group. As Dr Lourdes goes through Deirdre's current situation, I count off the other factors that have been identified as specifically risky in published case series of COVID patients: age, weight, history of high blood pressure, and the fact that she's spent a relatively long time on the ventilator, already six days. On the other hand, she is female and Caucasian, both seemingly "good" factors in the same literature. Dr Lourdes thinks she is brewing another infection, though. When we look through her blood results, nearly every line is red, denoting an abnormality. Her blood tests are incredibly deranged – liver function, kidney function, inflammatory markers. One of her blood markers, the D-dimer, is the highest I've ever seen, and has gone off the scale of what the lab can measure, so they've just left it as ">80 mg/L". I've never seen a result higher than 5 mg/L before this.

Dr Lourdes spends some time trying to get Deirdre's breathing better, umming and ahhing at the ventilator screen, slightly changing the settings to improve gas exchange. As she's doing that, she asks me to examine the patient. I don another plastic gown over the top of the first one and look for the bedside stethoscope, wiping it down carefully with an alcohol wipe before use. It's very hard to listen over the ventilator but I can hear her lungs crackle and bubble – more so on the right than the left. A new infection does seem likely.

"Let's discuss her antibiotics with microbiology," Dr Lourdes says.

"What shall I tell the family?" the SHO asks as she is typing into the computer on wheels.

"The same as before; she remains critically unwell."

I "doff" (remove) the plastic gown and we change our gloves-over-gloves between patients and apply alcohol gel to them.

I notice that my wrist has become exposed, and the nakedness feels odd, vulnerable even; the virus is invisible, yet I can almost imagine a fine weight settling on my bare skin. Just as quickly, I replace the gloves, tape them up and we are back.

The rest of the round in here is depressingly similar:

"Fifty years old, COVID pneumonia day 6, respiratory failure…"

"Sixty-four years old, COVID pneumonia day 7, respiratory failure…"

"Forty-eight years old, COVID pneumonia day 4, respiratory failure…"

I'm shocked by how young most of the patients are – only Deirdre is over 70. Except for Deirdre, all of the patients are male and from Asian or Afro-Caribbean backgrounds. It's unnerving how uniform the patients' conditions are; it's genuinely difficult to keep their parameters and stories separate. Last week, we had no patients on the unit, and now we have six. I wonder where we will be in a week's time or in two weeks as we finish the round and exit the bay, removing the PPE we just put on. It's a delicate dance, trying to make sure we don't accidentally touch the outer parts of the garments, possibly infecting ourselves even as we throw all the kit away. We wash our hands, and we are once again whisked away to do some ventilator training.

•   •   •

The programme for inducting doctors into ICU is impressive already, even at the inception of this new era. Like so many of the staff, the ICU team has been working around the clock to disseminate their vital skills to others as efficiently as possible, even if it's just the basics. It's something they will have to repeat dozens of times.

In our group, we run through a simulation of a patient assessment, shuffling around a plastic dummy attached to a monitor and an ICU ventilator. The group includes Helen, an oncology registrar, as well as some of the other doctors on training today. I only recognize my colleague Hugo, who is looking pretty pained to be here. I don't get a chance to say hello before the session begins. It feels a lot like medical school again – the training is rudimentary, enough to make us safe. The overriding and reassuring message of ventilator training is: "Don't touch the ventilator", followed by "Press the emergency button and call a senior or airway specialist". The simulation is reassuring – the ICU team understands we aren't intensivists, and they are ready to help and support us. It's very touching. The camaraderie here, in the sunlight of the emptied training ward, buoys me.

I catch Hugo in mid-conversation with one of the other intensive care doctors I don't know well, Cole. They are talking about the Nightingale Hospital, a place I haven't heard of.

"What's a Nightingale hospital? Is it like the open wards?" I ask, oblivious to the announcements of the day.

"It's awesome. They are converting the Excel Centre in the Docklands into a 4,000-bed hospital. In days." Hugo says, his eyes lighting up. Hugo is normally the most cynical person I know – it's odd to see him so energized by something, giddy even.

"How will they staff it?" I wonder out loud.

Hugo looks irritated at my perceived criticism.

"Us – you and me, Dom, and all the rest of London they are training, even beyond, I suppose. It's awesome." Hugo seems to remember something. "Didn't you say in that article of yours that we couldn't do something like this?"

I give a half-smile, remembering our argument about that article.

"You got me there – happy to be wrong about it." Genuinely, all I've ever wanted is to be wrong, about all of this. "It sounds epic."

"It does, doesn't it?" Hugo replies, pleased that I'm now sharing his enthusiasm. It certainly feels as if the cavalry is on the horizon.

. . .

On my break, I check my phone to catch up on what turns out to be frenetic activity on the charity front. Estée Lauder have donated 500 FFP masks, and we have arranged to get them to some local intensive care units in London. Meanwhile, the BBC have shown our video on air without crediting us and Jack is livid, but on the plus side, Joe Cole has rallied a whole host of England footballers to big up the charity on their socials. Michelle's contact hasn't got very far with the Cabinet at all, and the 30 million masks in China have been bought up by another country. In the midst of ITU, the calls for PPE that we are hearing feel all the more real – it's really grating to think of colleagues facing the same thing without protection. It isn't clear exactly what has happened, but I plan to phone on the way home to find out a bit more.

Beck's now our head of PR, which is a massive job given that we're about to finally publish the finished White Cliffs of Dover video. Beck pings me the final cut. It's such a bizarre moment, to watch a thousand-foot video of myself, Dilsan and

Zach, Michelle and others, and our logo, projected onto an iconic landmark, just as I walk back into the intensive care unit for the afternoon ward round.

I finish the day early, but it takes a while to leave the hospital after changing out of the PPE and waiting for the shower (there's only one at the moment), and then it's a long journey home. I try to avoid the crowds and take the overground, which is mercifully a little emptier; perhaps the longer-distance commuters have packed up already. The sky is seared with pink when I finally get out the tube on the other end. When I reach home, the house is busy and loud, with both Beck and Dilsan on the phone and Zach trying to run over Ayla in his walker. Beck looks stressed, but Dilsan looks happy. I feel a little extraneous to the goings-on at home, if I'm honest, and sneak upstairs to shower and change again, still paranoid about bringing COVID home. We'd even talked about me living elsewhere, but settled on this halfway house of quarantining the area around the front door and washing immediately. I know at least two doctors at work who moved out to protect the vulnerable family members they live with.

We get the kids to bed, and sit down with a glass of wine to watch the Dover video again on the big screen.

"It's day six and it feels like season five of 'House of Cards' already," Dilsan quips, partly to break the slightly emotional mood.

We are all a little stunned by how quickly this is moving, but I suppose that's what we wanted. The mantra of the tech world turned on its head: move fast, save things.

• • •

We spend the next training day as the intensive care team proper, starting early in the handover room; with so many staff on training and on regular ward duty, the ward feels oddly crowded. We make our rounds again, and little has changed. I'm getting a bit more familiar with the clicks and buzzes of the patients' machines. Dr Lourdes asks us to assess the patients and then present each one as part of a formal round. It's very much how we worked when I was in ICU years ago, and it's an easy pattern to fall back into. I go over each section of the ward round proforma in detail, remembering the mantra of one of the ICU consultants I worked for previously: "Good ICU care is simply doing many small things properly, every single day." I keep that in mind as I work from top to bottom on each patient, checking eyes, tubes and lines, listening to the chest, lungs and stomach, checking catheters and dressings, the blood tests, the microbiology samples, the drug chart, the feeding regime, the position of the patient – the list is endless. Despite all the hugely advanced kit and complex interventions, in proper head-to-head trials,* only a few very small things have been shown to make a big difference to patients: feeding them, protecting them from ulcers, controlling blood sugar levels, keeping the patient head-up, checking sedation and pain medications are dosed properly, and preventing blood clots. Abdul doesn't move very much when we stop his sedating medications temporarily to assess him, which is a bad sign.

Deirdre is equally unchanged – her ventilator settings are stuck where they were yesterday and the level of carbon dioxide

---

* In which one possible treatment is directly compared to another

in her blood is very slightly worse. The mood around her bedside is sombre, and the nurses are as sceptical on her outlook as we are. But we persist.

At the end of the ward round, there isn't very much to do – just replacing a venous line for one patient in the COVID-positive bay. It's something I'm very familiar with from day-to-day cardiology and, keen to do something useful, I happily volunteer to do it. I wander off to locate some kit, and manage to get lost in the storeroom. Lizzie is the regular junior doctor on the ward, but, having worked in intensive care for nearly a year now, she is far from junior, much more experienced in fact than me and many of my colleagues coming onto the unit now, even if we are, on paper at least, more senior. She takes pity on me and helps me find the stuff, and accompanies me to do the line exchange. We don the full PPE again, but this time I'm conscious of the flimsy acetate eye film, which makes it hard to see what I'm doing. Over the top of the PPE, we put on sterile gloves and another gown, and I'm now oddly wearing three layers, and it's uncomfortably hot. This is a procedure I've done tens of times before, but new obstacles make it difficult, as I clamber among the lines and wires around the patient's head, trying to position myself to put in a suture and wire exchange. It's such a simple procedure, but seems to take an age and I struggle, embarrassingly, apologizing to Lizzie for making her watch such a clumsy procedure. When we are done, I'm sweating in three layers of PPE, and the nurses are laughing at the terrible dressing I've placed, but the line is in and working. I'm sure it'll get better. I hope.

I check in with home – the charity WhatsApp group is buzzing, as we've just passed £100,000 in donations. Candy

Kittens, the sweet company owned and run by "Made in Chelsea" star Jamie Laing, has offered to partner with us. On a more sombre note, Northwick Park hospital has reportedly nearly run out of FFP3 masks, and we are trying to see if we have any left to send them. It isn't clear if it's a supply issue or a logistics one. Supposedly the army is getting involved to help deliver kit to the NHS, but it isn't clear when this will happen. In the meantime, we try to think of ways to help. Michelle suggests novel ways to reuse stock and make it last, which gets me thinking.

I catch up with Dr Desmond about what the procurement here is like – what does the unit need in terms of masks and goggles? He seems interested in the idea of us producing visors, and is happy to try them on the ward. I ask him about the possibility of decontaminating some of the kit we are using. He shrugs before saying: "I'm not sure we have the facilities for that." I wonder if that's true.

I spend some of the afternoon looking up the effect of air and heat on coronavirus; it turns out it's not an especially robust virus, and completely disintegrates after 30 minutes in a 60°C oven, which is barely hot. There's a paper from the US that has just been published, which suggests that FFP masks can withstand the heat without breaking down and still retain their filtering function. In the afternoon break, I wander along the corridor to the now-disused kitchen between the wards; there's an oven in there, dialable up to 200°C and large enough to accommodate six trays. I take some pictures for later.

At the end of the day, it takes an hour to leave the hospital – to hand over, to get changed, to shower, and to get changed again. I'm so thirsty my mouth feels like cotton. I must keep hydrated, I try to remind myself. When I get home, Dilsan makes me strip and shower again. It's well past 11 p.m. by the time we're in bed. I sleep like the dead.

• • •

Despite not having a shift and feeling like death warmed up, I get up early the next morning (26 March). There is another potential TV interview at 8 a.m., but by 7.30 a.m. it gets cancelled again. I'm getting used to this by now, and at least we are up and about. There's plenty to be doing.

I spend the morning trying to do some reading up on intensive care, schooling myself on fluid management, dose of drugs to make the blood pressure and the heart function improve, ventilator settings and emergencies. It's a lot to learn and I find it hard to take it in, while also trying to spend some time with the kids. By mid-morning, I have a call with a 3D-printing professional, Dr Nate Petre, to discuss the manufacturing of reusable PPE, a novel idea. We set up a Zoom call and Nate pops into view; with his soft American accent and raffish flop of black hair, Nate is a real character, full of energy and enthusiasm. He is also oddly exactly qualified for responding to a pandemic; he has just written a PhD thesis on disseminated distributive manufacturing in a crisis, and previously worked for NASA, 3D-printing surfboards in Jamaica. He's calling me from Makerversity, a consortium of "makers" – engineers, designers and inventors, based in the historic Somerset House in London. As we chat, he wanders around the cavernous rooms.

"So the ideal way to create new stuff in a crisis would be to create one place with a whole ton of 3D printers, a 'print farm'," Nate drawls as we watch one of his 3D printers whip gracefully back and forth across a glass plate, laying thin lines of perfectly precise molten plastic. Slowly, the shape of a visor headband begins to emerge, rising off the plate. "You'd only need one 'farmer', to run the place," he tells me. This sounds like a great, efficient way to use the funds.

"And how many printers can you get in there?"

"Mmm…" Nate looks around. "One hundred–200?"

"And how many visors could that make – 2,000?"

"Up to 6,000 if we really pushed it."

"A week?" I ask.

Nate laughs. "No, a day."

This seems really encouraging. I ask Nate to draw up some plans and we think about how to get the farm going. He promises to get me some prototypes to try in ICU that weekend.

• • •

That afternoon I feel antsy, itchy. Needing something constructive to occupy my mind, I decide to put one of the industrial FFP3 masks we have at home in the oven, following the instructions in the US study, and check the fit before and after. I get Beck to help me make a little video of them for Twitter. Ayla thinks it's hilarious. It seems to work reasonably well. Michelle checks in – her ICU is in full COVID swing now, but she's noticed more than a few swollen eyes around and wonders when the counselling services we're providing will be coming online. We hope by the weekend. In the meantime, new ambassadors are joining us. I hear that Elton John is thinking of donating, we are hopefully going to be on "Good Morning Britain" and

"BBC Breakfast" in the morning, and there's a prototype visor to pick up.

That evening, we are sitting discussing food drops and PPE budgets over the kitchen table. Beck checks her phone and stands up.

"C'mon," she says. "Time for this clapping for carers thing."

I read about this on Twitter in the last few days, and, if I'm honest, am not sure what the point is. It seems like a silly thing and I'm not sure anyone will even buy into it, so I haven't given it too much attention. I hadn't planned on going outside at 8 p.m. at all. There's frankly quite a lot to do otherwise, to say the least.

"No, Dom. C'mon," Beck says, tugging on my arm. Dilsan follows us out too.

As we get closer to the door, there's an odd sound I haven't really heard before, a blunted pattering like the sound of distant rain on wood.

"What is that?" I ask.

We open the door to the sight of everyone on our street, on their doorsteps, clapping. The sound of the applause echoes from streets away. Our immediate neighbours, Mariella and Victor, are on their drive, and turn to us as we come out as well, clapping and hollering.

I really didn't know what I expected – lockdown has only really just started and everyone is feeling isolated, alone. This sudden burst of connection, the sense of togetherness in the face of adversity, the acknowledgement of the mutual effort, not just in the NHS, I find overwhelming. Somewhat embarrassed, I'm tearing up and sniffling, and so is Beck behind me. We're clapping as well, for my colleagues and my friends, for all of those doing so much to help in the pandemic. It's heart-warming. And then, just like that, it's over. We are all rubbing tears from our cheeks as we walk back through the door. Beck breaks the silence.

"Wine?"

. . .

Early the following morning, I receive confirmation that the interviews on both "Good Morning Britain" and "BBC Breakfast" are going ahead, back to back. I've never actually met Joe Cole in real life, or even spoken to him up to that point except via intermediaries, so appearing side-by-side via Skype a couple of hours later was another of so many surreal experiences of the pandemic. On both shows, Joe is a natural ambassador for us, and really expresses the true values of what we are trying to do, far better than I can. He talks passionately and simply about the charity on the television – he really gets it. I stick to our agreed line, to create positive action, highlighting our wish to help the government and harness that goodwill of everyone doing their bit. Unlike my previous TV appearance, I feel fine during the interview but light-headed and sick afterwards. Nerves, I suppose. The feedback is good, and the emails are flooding in already. Nikki Lovell of Flavour Management, who represents celebratory chefs including Tony Singh, Francesco Mazzei and Aldo Zilli, has just seen us on television and really wants to get involved in the charity. One of her chefs, Omar Allibhoy, wants to make paella for the NHS today. We spend the day trying to connect him to his local hospital, and get some really satisfying photos of doctors and nurses enjoying some top-restaurant-quality food that afternoon. Everyone just wants to help.

Around lunchtime all my groups light up with the same news. Boris Johnson has reportedly tested positive for coronavirus. It's hardly surprising, as among journalists and cabinet MPs (ironically, the groups who should be the most informed), the virus has been particularly rampant. Boris was boasting of "shaking hands with everybody" only three weeks ago. Last week, I tweeted that they should probably stop "in-the-room" press conferences given how much COVID appeared to be spreading around Westminster, and now here we are. As one of my colleagues puts it, "Human male is diagnosed with highly infectious disease", but it's still jarring, however, and I genuinely dread to think what could happen if he gets seriously sick with it. Reportedly, the Health Secretary and the Chief Medical Officer have been diagnosed as well. It makes an impact, especially among the non-medics we know. If there were a message to tell the country to take this seriously, this is it.

But the work is in front of us – Northwick Park has run out of visors as well as gowns. Rumours abound that senior colleagues are on ventilators all over London. I pick up a prototype visor from Nate – it's sturdy and robust, and far better than the ones we are already using. I wonder if it can be disinfected. That evening I'm on a night shift, so I try to get some sleep in the afternoon, although without much success. I struggle to convince my body that it needs to sleep when my brain is still running at a hundred miles an hour, stretching itself in too many directions, too fast. The manic energy is keeping me going – if I stop, it feels like I will sink. It's hard to switch that off, even to rest. After a couple of hours of tossing and turning, I get up again, shower, and get ready for work.

· · ·

The journey to work at dusk is warm and strange. The underground is, finally, blissfully deserted. Friday night, going in the opposite direction to the commuter crowd, I would've expected it to be quiet, but in the end I don't see a soul for five stops. I sit and write some notes and plans for the charity – we've already expanded to over 15 people and more are coming in. There's reams of emails and messages to catch up on. By the time I look up, I'm at the tube station and out. Everything is closed – all the restaurants and shops. I forgot to bring any food and left the house without eating. It's an odd moment experiencing a sense of food insecurity – I've never really felt it before. It's going to be a long shift if I can't find anything to eat. Mercifully, a Tesco is still open, and I get some supplies.

Hospitals seem to take on properties of time and space all of their own now. Each time I go back to work, time has stuttered forward with sudden staccato changes, without any gradation in between. I find that a ward has moved, or closed, or is sealed, or is COVID only, or is COVID "clean". The lockers fly around the hospital like they are alive, moving from changing room to changing room. I've already lost my theatre shoes since that second day in ICU, and I don't expect to see them again anytime soon.

We are now running a parallel rota system, involving two sets of shift patterns: one for the original cardiology rota of wards and clinics; and the new "COVID" rotas, where we're working on COVID wards or in intensive care. Watching the rota evolve is a marvel in itself; the incredible amount of work that has fallen on the rota leads is only surpassed by the effort they are putting into it daily in order to master it. The spreadsheet is a thing of beauty, of streams of colour and order, that changes each day as new registrars and juniors jump onto the rota. It's hard to keep up with.

Right now, I'm in an odd limbo between my old job and intensive care. I was due to move into intensive care properly, except for three sequential "standby" nights over the weekend to cover for colleagues if they fall ill themselves or have reason to self-isolate. The rules are still fairly stringent, and we don't have routine testing yet, meaning a few colleagues have been forced to stay home wondering whether they have COVID or not. I'd crossed my fingers, hoping for a free weekend, but, inevitably, it isn't. I got the call this morning – someone's sick and I need to cover the COVID ward overnight. The hospitalized patients are usually sick enough that they need oxygen or even a ventilator, such as those very sick patients in intensive care, but we also have patients who are not unwell enough with COVID-19 to warrant being in hospital normally, but who have come in with other things, like heart attacks or dysfunctional or infected heart valves that require surgery. In the ward, there are only a handful of patients with COVID who are completely well, their surgery or other heart treatments being delayed while they remain positive. The active instruction is to keep as safe as possible, and "do not see the patients" unless we genuinely really have to. So, we conduct overnight remote reviews, carefully going through their observations and their notes, and hand over again in the morning to the day team. Each night I read their stories, these patients with coronavirus, and never see their faces.

The first patient is a young woman transferred to consider for heart-valve surgery. She has an infected heart valve, with a clump of bacteria sitting on the main valve leaving her heart, the aortic valve. The COVID swab taken when she was admitted turned up positive, despite her having no real symptoms. All patients coming into hospital are getting "swabbed" now when they land, which involves inserting a long stick of plastic with a cotton bud on the end up the nose and to the back of the mouth. It's deeply unpleasant, and if the patient doesn't gag on it, you aren't doing it properly. The big problem is that it seems the current swabs miss about one-third of all positive cases, meaning we can't be sure that the negative swabs indicate that the patient truly is coronavirus-free. There are several patients in intensive care with what appears to be severe COVID pneumonia that have had multiple negative swab tests. We aren't really sure why – perhaps we aren't doing the swabs properly, or maybe some patients don't have sufficient virus in their throat and mouth to detect. It makes "cohorting" patients into positive and negative groups difficult.

The next patient has had a heart attack, coming in with chest pain and a big change in her blood markers of heart damage, troponins. I look through her coronary angiogram pictures, the grey and white 2D films of dye being injected into each coronary artery. The junior doctor on shift with me, Gregoris, sucks the air through his teeth when he sees her pictures. Her arteries are so narrowed and calcified they resemble gnarled tree roots, strictured and irregular from end to end and critically narrow in several places. She might need surgery but developed a mild cough on arrival and had contact with a coronavirus patient in the same bay at another hospital and has now tested positive herself. I wonder if the coronavirus patient was any of the ones I have seen over the last few weeks, but by now we have probably hundreds of cases in London, and it seems very unlikely. Nearly fully recovered from her heart attack and waiting for a surgical review, again she is just waiting.

We come to the end of the list. Normally we would be covering the whole hospital overnight, but as we are still trying to keep the COVID-19 patients away from everyone else, that means separate teams as well. We have nowhere to go, and, for now, very little to do but be present in case anything is needed. Gregoris and I chat a little; he is planning on applying for a training job in cardiology here in the UK and he picks my brain about my experience. I reassure him that he is already halfway there, with his experience here, and highlight the importance of the interview. As we talk, I realize that there may not even be interviews this year due to COVID, or perhaps they will conduct them online. Everybody's lives are being disrupted so fundamentally.

When we finish chatting, I look at the clock. It's still only 10 p.m. I feel restless again, that manic energy with nowhere to go trapped in the on-call room. I try to work on my other life, the charity, overnight to fill the time, reaching out to a few other charity groups. Two former peers of mine are running two other initiatives themselves. They're an enterprising bunch, and it's good to catch up and swap notes on their approaches. As the night drags on, I try to get some sleep in the on-call room but can't seem to get the temperature right. Usually we'd be able to go down to the mess, but this is a restricted area now and so that just isn't possible. The night passes without incident.

On the Saturday morning, I stay up to plug the charity – which now has expanded to 30 people – on "The Nigel Farage Show" on LBC radio, giving a dozy interview but managing to mention the charity at least twice. I get some sleep during the day, then head back out. Meanwhile, the ward, like a time-lapse movie, fills up exponentially, and each night, I return to a significantly higher number of cases. By the end of the weekend, they have to close this ward entirely to make room for more intensive care beds and open another COVID ward elsewhere for the well patients. The hospital is continuously reconfiguring. On the Sunday night, the patients are transferred downstairs, and by Monday morning, it's all changed again.

We are only seeing the tip of the iceberg here, the overflow from other hospitals which have been overwhelmed. I hear of surgical theatres being converted to new COVID ventilation areas and nearly entire hospitals being given over to treat COVID patients only. They're struggling to keep up with the pressure on oxygen supplies, the demand for beds and the required staffing levels. We are hurtling downhill and there's no end in sight.

* * *

On the Monday, we move into a three/four shift pattern, working long 13-hour shifts in three- or four-day runs, with three or four days' recovery, and then repeat. I stay up that day, trying to catch up with the charity. Tamara Ecclestone and her husband Jay Rutland are becoming ambassadors and are announcing the initiative Art for Heroes at the Maddox Gallery in Mayfair, which looks to catapult our fundraising to another level. I haven't heard anything back from the Cabinet Office about the large-scale PPE purchases from abroad, so I give them a call. They are waiting on more paperwork, so I ping Michelle and her contact and try to expedite things. Strangely enough, the PPE suppliers' UK base is only five minutes from my front door, so I wonder about going directly to their premises. It's really hard to listen to all the pockets of need around the country coming to us via the charity and its links and to know that the solution could be just a freight-plane away, if only we can connect the dots.

Worried about the upcoming ICU shifts at the weekend again, I message one of the best doctors I've ever worked with, Mac. An intensive care registrar now, we were SHOs together when I did ICU the first time around. He would routinely blow every other doctor on the unit out of the water with his outlandish and yet totally accurate diagnoses, including cancers or infections that senior doctors had missed, far beyond his level at the time. I tried to glean as much as I could from Mac back then, and heading back into ICU now, thought I'd see if he could send me any tips.

"Can you teach me to do intensive care? 280 characters or less, please," I jokingly message him.

His response is pitch-perfect, and comes back nearly instantly.

"Gas goes in and out, blood goes round and round."

This becomes a mantra I say to myself over and over in the coming months. As I'm messaging Mac, another message pops into my inbox, from Hugo. He opens in typically blunt fashion, referencing the argument we had a few weeks ago.

"Okay, you were right. We're f**ked," he says, his tone a far cry from his former hardened scepticism.

I try to be conciliatory. "It'll be okay, Hugo. When are you starting in ICU? I'm in on the weekend."

"Hoping to go to the Nightingale." Hugo did seem pumped about it the last time we spoke, and it would be a good place to transfer to.

"Let me know how it goes."

"Will do."

I stretch out the morning with one more meeting; I have been connecting all the PPE groups together for a regular video call and have been helping to combine their logistics and procurement expertise. It's a really satisfying process, with a Zoom gallery that seems to double in size every day. Between Paul, Michelle and I, we are connecting engineers, designers, 3D printers, volunteers, other doctors – everyone wants to work together. We plan to build a 3D print farm in London, which Nate is working on, and potentially another near Manchester. These hubs need a name, though. Nate knows I like acronyms and suggests: Sustainable Hubs for Innovative Emergent Local Development (SHIELD). Dilsan is less than pleased that I've started a whole other organization. My life is getting so hectic already, I really need some help.

I put a call out on Twitter for a PA and the very first respond-ent is a post-doctoral physicist called Dr Jess Wade. She's super motivated, willing to help with anything we need, and comes from a family of doctors.

"Oh, anyone we might know?" I ask during our initial chat over Zoom.

"Well, my brother is an F2 (second-year doctor) in London and my dad is a neurologist."

"Hold on, is your dad Dr John Wade?" I ask.

"Yes! Do you know him?"

John Wade was the only neurologist at the hospital that both Dilsan and I started working at in our very first year. We would knock nervously on his door each week with whatever nonsense referral had been sent to him. He probably wouldn't remember us, but he was a key thread in the tapestry of that formative year.

We laugh at the coincidence. Jess is already practically family. She's in, and instantly brings some organization and some great ideas to the table.

We spend the week organizing to set up the London print farm, our first SHIELD hub. We are trying to organize food trucks, and a coffee stall where the coffee shop in a hospital has closed down. There's always more and more to do.

Beck and Dilsan are stressed – the charity has become a fire that is burning bigger and bigger, and it feels like every time I come back from the hospital, I throw more oil on it. Increasingly, I'm leaving it to them, and Rosh and Nej. There's a backlog of people to manage, of website goals to sort, of relationships to follow up on. It was always going to be like this – we are trying to help in a pandemic, a problem so vast it would never feel like any level of effort was enough. Beck is finding it particularly tough. She came here to rest from her already hectic life, not to run teams of marketing people. She hasn't balked or backed away. It's a lot to ask of anyone, and we've had more than a few fights over tiny things this week already. A guilty part of me wonders whether this is really worth it after all; what have I dragged us all into?

By mid-week, things are starting to take shape with SHIELD. I get a message on Twitter from a friend of mine, working in a hospice. Her message sounds distraught:

"Dear Dom, I'm sorry to bother you when you are probably 1,000 per cent too busy, but I am desperate… my hospice is on the brink of having to close the entire inpatient unit because we cannot get surgical masks from anywhere. We've tried the emergency NHS COVID supply chain people, even tried all our local vets, but the NHS aren't helping us and we can't keep staff and patients safe (we have suspected cases here) so may have to close completely by this weekend. I'm not sure if you have funds for PPE, but can I possibly beg for some masks? Just asking out of sheer desperation."

I hadn't realized the hospice situation was so dire, and so ignored outside of the regular NHS infrastructure. And, thinking about it, of course it is an area that is going to struggle with PPE, just like care homes, even funeral homes. I don't want to overpromise anything, though, so I simply reply "I'll see what we can do". I call up Paul Ford from Contractors Appeal and explain the situation.

"Is there any way we can help?"

Paul responds in his typical fashion.

"Yes, will sort."

And that's it. I connect my friend and Paul, and she messages me later that afternoon.

"Dom!!! Paul can deliver 1,000 masks tomorrow. I literally burst into tears on the phone. I cannot tell you how grateful we all are – just thank you, a million times."

My voice cracks on the evening call with the whole team to tell them about this. We haven't really done anything, just connected the dots, but now a hospice is open this weekend when it might not otherwise have been. Perhaps it is all worth it after all.

* * *

The next evening – 2 April – it's Thursday again and coming to that 8 p.m. clapping time. I'm knackered, having already given an interview to ITV that evening about the charity. Weirdly, the segment follows a story about mass mortuaries being built in London, which is filmed from a spot on my own street using a new socially distanced television technique.

As moving as I found the clapping for carers the week before, I don't think it would be repeatable, and that previous cynicism has returned. I wonder how long this will last. Beck drags me outside again regardless, and as that same wave of sounds hits me, seeing all the neighbours on the street, hearing the claps on social media coming over the flats and houses of all parts of the country, I'm teary-eyed all over again. For us, it's not just a clap for the NHS, it's a clap for everyone that's trying to do their bit, whether that's Nesli and Ehsan locking away for months, the general public doing the same, the Paul Fords and Michelle Dawsons of the world, or all of the rest, giving their all in a moment of crisis to make life better for their fellow human beings, even if just by a tiny bit.

. . .

The next morning, I'm heading back into my next run of intensive care shifts. Dilsan is keen that I try to avoid public transport, so I drive in. I use the time to catch up with Nej on the car phone. Parking is free around the hospital now, and driving on empty streets through central London as the early morning sun is slanting through the high-rises is actually quite relaxing. I wonder if road traffic accidents must be on the decline during lockdown, given the complete lack of cars around. I tuck the car into a local car park and find that all the barriers are up – it feels like it's been abandoned. It's a short, cold walk to the hospital. Nothing is open. I kick myself for not making a coffee at home. Not a good way to start my first proper shift as an intensive care doctor. As I approach the building, I realize I've returned to a changed hospital again. This time the main gates are closed, and I have to pick my way through a side entrance to get in, eventually following a pair of likely-looking staff to find where we need to go.

The floors have been rearranged and I can't get into the door to the changing area now. We've moved to "sessional" use for PPE, which means we wear the same PPE for the whole shift, without donning and doffing between patients' rooms. It also implies the entire ward is "dirty" now, not just the patient rooms but their surroundings, the desks and the walls, the computers, the pens and the office. It is eerie to think of COVID being everywhere. In several studies in China they reported randomly swabbing parts of a hospital with COVID patients, and finding that one-third of these swabs came back positive with samples of the virus. I remember this paper well, because Dilsan texted it to me, with the subtitle "One-third of swans tested positive". I remember thinking, oh God, that's all we need, swans as well as cats and bats and whatever other animal vectors are out there. But then her additional "*swabs" text underneath clarified the mistake. My brain clearly was ready to believe the worst about the virus, however ridiculous it sounded in retrospect. Even so, it showed it to be an incredibly resilient and sticky virus on surfaces.

I have this in mind as I don the PPE downstairs, slightly more experienced now and following the tips I've copied from some of the nurses, like cutting a little hole into each sleeve cuff to slip your thumb through, keeping the sleeves from rolling up and exposing the wrist. I'm learning to write my name on my chest when wearing the gown, which isn't easy given that the writing needs to be both upside-down and back-to-front. I'm shocked we are still so profligate in disposing of so much, though. The eyewear I find particularly irksome. Someone has furnished the department with hundreds of pairs of swimmers' goggles, but they are tight, hot and uncomfortable to wear for hours. It's also hard to clean them. Luckily, I've brought one of Nate's prototype visors in today to test out on the unit; it's airy and durable and feels like a helmet when I put it on. I find myself thinking of an adapted line from the film *Full Metal Jacket*: "This is my visor, there are many like it, but this one is mine".

There are different masks in the ICU today – there's a hard type of industrial-looking mask with a valve, not one I've seen before, with a metal mouldable band over the nose. As I squeeze it down to make the fit, I notice lots of the staff are bringing in adhesive padding to prevent sores where the mask digs in over the nose. I make a mental note to get some for myself. We don the gear and take another lift upstairs. I bump into a junior doctor I worked my first shift in intensive care with, Lizzie, in the donning room – she is working with me this weekend, and the presence of someone familiar and so experienced is a huge relief.

The lockdown is well under way at this point, and it's been weeks since I shook a hand or made physical contact with another person outside my household. The night registrar handing over this morning is another cardiology colleague, Denise, and I offer her my double-gloved and gowned hand as a greeting. She takes it and we shake hands in full PPE, feeling far more awkward about a handshake than we are about wearing all the layers of kit. We both give a little laugh before getting on with handing the patients over. Dr Desmond is the consultant again. Having the same team makes a big difference, and I wonder why we don't try and organize into "firms" like this for the duration.

As with every shift now, after a gap of more than a few days, everything is exponentially different. This unit is now full, as is the additional intensive care unit that has been assembled next door. Every patient has the same diagnosis, "COVID pneumonia", but they've had varying numbers of days on the ventilator, each of them requires different levels of heart, kidney and lung support, and a few have acquired new bacterial infections. Some of the patients have already been on ventilators for more than two weeks now, and several patients aren't doing well at all.

Listening to the patients' stories, it seems like the more we know about COVID-19, the less we really know. The basics are unchanged for now, however: COVID-19 is a virus, comprising tiny particles of genetic material wrapped in an envelope of protein, the whole package called a virion. These pass from person to person through the air or on surfaces, and land on the exposed linings of the nose or mouth, where they can enter the cells and take over the cellular mechanics to start making more virions. There is some debate over whether or not viruses are actually alive, in the same way we would consider other micro-organisms to be; on the tiniest level they are like microscopic machines, unpacking their blueprints into cells they land on, in order to replicate more of the virus. The presence of the virus in these cells causes damage to them, and the body to react to them as foreign material, attacking the cells and causing the inflammation and irritation at the site. The virus has been reported to be able to get to many parts of the body, mostly the airways and lungs, but also the heart, the bowels and even the brain.

It takes some time after catching the virus, called exposure, to actually start manifesting symptoms, a period of time we call the "incubation" period, with the latest reports ranging from a few days up to two weeks. This is partly due to the time it takes for the virus to replicate in sufficient quantities to cause symptoms, which implies a higher "level" of virus present at the moment that symptoms are produced,* which may be linked to how likely you are to infect others. Right now, we don't really understand why, but when the virus passes from person

* https://www.nature.com/articles/s41591-020-0869-5

to person they can react very differently, a spectrum from no symptoms at all, to merely a mild dry cough, fever, fatigue or lack of smell or taste, all the way to severe pneumonia, heart muscle inflammation, kidney failure, blood clots and death. Other symptoms, like diarrhoea, headache and muscle pain, also seem to occur occasionally. The virus "sheds" into the nose and mouth, as well as into faeces,* which is how it can be transferred to others, either directly or via contaminated surfaces, including your hands. The bad news is how long-lived it can be, as it can now reportedly survive on surfaces for up to three days† and is still able to infect others. The good news, however, is that it appears to be easily disrupted with alcohol gel, soap, and even gentle heat.

The patients needing intensive care are on the severest end of the spectrum, their lungs criss-crossed with patchy areas of inflamed lung, filled with pus and the surrounding soft aerated lung scarred into hardened knots of useless tissue. The commonest presentation in hospitals is cough and fever. Weirdly, we've seen many patients come in with very low oxygen but not reporting they feel at all short of breath, and it's only when we perform tests that we find a dangerous, life-threateningly low level of oxygen in the blood. Again, no one seems to know why this is happening.

From what we can see in the wards at the moment, there seem to be distinct phases to severe COVID-19 infection, a short period of perhaps a week of slowly worsening symptoms

---

* And even reportedly in sperm, although it isn't clear if that means it can be sexually transmitted
† https://www.nejm.org/doi/full/10.1056/nejmc2004973

and then a crashing illness for a few days, and then most stabilize, not quite getting better but not really getting worse, in that critical zone on the edge of catastrophe. Sometimes they can unpredictably lose oxygenation after days of improvement, as a result of an extreme lung inflammatory reaction called Acute Respiratory Distress Syndrome. The presence of fluid in the tiny bubbles of lung tissue called alveoli interrupts the normal exchange of gas between inhaled air and the blood, meaning oxygen can't get in and carbon dioxide can't get out. Over time, the lungs appear to stiffen and harden, the soft, delicate, sponge-like tissue scarring into thick blocks that move less and less, requiring more and more pressure to move air in and move air out again. This plateau phase seems to stretch on and on, a dark tunnel from which, so far, we have seen few come out.

Most of the patients on the ward had symptoms for a week or more before needing a ventilator. What we "know" about the virus seems to change nearly weekly; some advocate for putting patients on an invasive ventilator earlier, while others say prolonging other types of simple ventilation that can be managed without patients needing to be paralyzed and unconscious might be better. There's no time for the thorough processes of trial and science that we would usually use to answer some of these questions properly, though, and we are operating on the best information from a series of cases and anecdotes as we go. Trials are starting up at a blistering pace, but it's still too slow to be useful today.

Many patients also seem to run into trouble with their kidneys at a similar time. Firstly, they stop making urine, and then further fluid builds up in the body, as well as all the toxic waste-products that can't be safely excreted, leading to a dangerous build-up of salts that can cause a whole host of deadly complications without rapid rectification using a kidney-replacement machine. We are seeing far too many problems with blood clots, too, and begin to wonder if that's the virus as well, causing clots in machine circuits, in legs and in lungs.

At first, COVID-19 looks like the most bizarre disease any of us has seen before, but I wonder if that's down to the sheer volume of patients. Almost any disease will have an accompanying list, in small print, of the rarest complications that have been reported in 1 in 10,000 or perhaps 1 in 100,000 of those infected. But what would happen if the world saw millions of cases of any disease all at once? We would see all of those "rare" side-effects with increasing regularity. And our view is entirely skewed in intensive care, as we don't see any of the thousands if not tens of thousands of patients with mild or no symptoms – just the ones with present symptoms. Close up, and in great numbers, any disease process might look as bizarre, with so much uncertainty. Like looking at a fingernail under a high-powered microscope, what we had perceived to be a flat and smooth surface is actually a ridged terrain of dizzying peaks and deep troughs. It's all a matter of perspective, I suppose.

As I listen to handover, itchy and uncomfortably warm in full PPE, so many of the patients here sound like they are stuck in that dark tunnel of the plateau phase. After handover, Dr Desmond divides the patients between me and Lizzie to review and hares off to chair a meeting of the hospital network, his mobile phone buzzing already. There are some sheepish white-clad doctors lurking around outside the handover room, the next batch of doctors to be cross-trained standing where I was only a week ago. Lizzie and I divide them between us and take them to see the patients.

There's a glib catchphrase in medicine: "See one, do one, teach one". I've seen one, done one, and now here I am "teaching" one. My apprentice for the morning is Chloe, a junior doctor from oncology, only qualified for a year and a half, who has never been in intensive care before. I show her the ropes as we see our first patient, and I'm acutely aware that the ropes are only slightly more familiar to me than to her.

Ali is a 67-year-old florist, still running his own flower shop until just four weeks ago. He'd had a cough and a fever that had lingered for days, and, despite his protestations, he ended up in his local A&E two weeks ago, where they'd found that his blood oxygen levels were far too low. It's such a typical story. Within two days Ali had to be put onto a ventilator and then was transferred here.

Chloe reads out the handover notes:

"Day 15 COVID pneumonia," Chloe starts. Normally, two weeks unconscious on a ventilator, with a tube splinting open the vocal cords and blowing air into the lungs, is a long time, so we might consider instead putting in a different tube directly into the base of the neck (a tracheostomy), which is far more comfortable and means that the patient requires little or no sedation, so we have the option of waking them up. There's currently some debate over whether or not we should perform a tracheostomy in COVID patients at all – the risk of aerosolizing the virus as the tracheostomy ventilates is possibly dangerous, and we still don't know if it's the right thing to do.

We go through the process of examining and recording Ali, from top to toe. We see if his pupils respond to light and check the length of the tube at the mouth. I have a listen with the bedside stethoscope to his heart sounds and bowel sounds. His lungs crackle with each breath of the ventilator on both sides. We examine his legs, check the sites of the intravenous lines in his wrist and neck and note down how long they've been in. From the bedside, among the whirs and ticks of the ventilator and the soft beeping of the infusion pumps, he looks stable, paralyzed to help him breathe better and deeply asleep on a cocktail of drugs.

The numbers tell a different story, revealing a slow downward trend in the amount of oxygen in his blood and a trickling rise in the carbon dioxide levels, so more and more ventilation is required. He's been stable for days, although unable to come down from his ventilator settings, but now he seems to be slipping down a steeper precipice. It's not looking good for him.

"Has he had any family come in?" Chloe asks the bedside nurse, whose PPE badge reads "Kayla, ICU nurse". Very sensibly, the nurses have written their full roles as well, as we can't recognize anyone under the layers of visors and masks, even if we know each other by face, which, in an ever-expanding unit, is very unlikely. In turn, I've written, "Dom, Cardio SpR"* on my PPE, to clearly delineate myself from the proper ICM-trained registrars around. In an emergency this makes a real difference.

Kayla shakes her head.

"No, no family visits allowed." Her voice is a little muffled, as are all of ours. "Only staff allowed up here now."

---

* Specialist registrar

This makes sense – every surface of the ward is potentially infected, it's too dangerous to bring healthy relatives up every day, and we don't have the PPE supplies to manage that anyway. Daily visits are another casualty of the pandemic, sadly, but Chloe is slightly perturbed by this.

"What, no visits AT ALL?" she asks, disbelievingly. The idea of a ward without relatives, especially in the afternoon when they are ubiquitous in every other part of the hospital, is totally alien, to all of us.

"Well, only if the patient is dying," Kayla explains. "You know, to say goodbye."

This grim thought hits like a soft thump in the chest. It's a dark start to the morning, especially as I wonder when we should think about these types of conversations with Ali's family.

"There is a system, though," Kayla adds, perhaps trying to buoy Chloe's spirits. "The families can call and I think they have a tablet to video-call the patients, although I'm not sure it's working yet."

Dr Desmond joins us at the bedside, looking slightly harassed. We've heard that other hospitals are having to close their A&Es and other departments, that they're running out of oxygen, with patients overflowing into theatres and outpatient wards to keep up with the deluge. All of them are calling here for beds, beds, beds.

"Tell us the story, Dom," Dr Desmond asks me.

I relay the history again and our assessment for Dr Desmond, a practice known in medicine as "presenting". "Presenting" is a lot harder than it looks at first; it takes years to sieve what is and isn't relevant information for a colleague, and to learn how to precisely and concisely relay that in a sensible way for them to digest. It's a big part of our medical school exams. As I start presenting, it feels like one of those strange throwback moments, where I'm back before the examiner, stumbling through unfamiliar terrain again as I try to get all the parameters and assessments in a sensible order. Dr Desmond is clearly pained but impressively patient as he listens, without interruption. He is an excellent trainer and it shows.

"Okay, so what's your plan?" he asks me.

If I'm honest, I don't really have one. There's nowhere to go once the patient is on the ventilator, no medicines or treatments we could add.

Dr Desmond can see I'm struggling, frowning at the latest blood gas analysis.

"We should prone him," he says over the top of the report.

. . .

Right now, we have few options when it comes to treating COVID-19. From some wider reading, I know there are ongoing trials of antiviral medicines, the potential to use steroids to dampen the immune response and even infusions of vitamins to potentially do the same. The debate about anti-malarial drugs, like hydroxychloroquine, rages back and forth, unhelpfully dipped into by politicians and profiteering companies. A vaccine is a distant horizon though. Our treatment is essentially supportive, as one of the consultants puts it, "as that's what all intensive care really is". We can keep oxygen levels up and kidneys going, react to bacterial infections and low fluids – but ultimately the virus burns away unhindered, until the body can get on top of it and start to heal. For some, this is nothing more than a minor cough, or even no symptoms at all, and for others, this can mean weeks and months in intensive care in multi-organ failure – we are yet to work out why some people are affected so severely.

The one "treatment" that does seem to help the very sickest patients is a technique called "proning". Normally, intensive care patients are nursed and ventilated on their backs, which makes sense; this gives easy access to examine them, to the breathing tube, to put in and access lines in the neck and groin, and keeps their face free to the air and identifiable. Intensive care is already one of the most dehumanizing environments in the modern world – turning the patient over to hide their face only exacerbates this. But that is exactly what we are going to do for Ali – flip him over with his lines, tubes and all, to lie on his front. The exact physiology of why we do this I struggle to understand. Dr Desmond is kind to me, and deploys a technique known in the medical game as "teaching by proxy" – i.e. to spare my blushes, he directs his questions to the most junior team member, Chloe.

"Do you know how proning improves oxygenation?" he asks Chloe, who simply shakes her head.

We go and find a whiteboard, and, thank goodness, Dr Desmond keeps it simple.

"Okay, here are two sets of lungs," he says, putting up a simple diagram of a pair of lungs.

"Gas goes in and out, blood goes round and round." I nearly laugh to hear this again, but it is a very simple way to explain the two key parts of getting oxygen into the blood – air needs to go back and forth through the lungs, into ever smaller and smaller branches until it reaches the alveoli, bubbles of tissue just a few microns in size, where oxygen can diffuse across a membrane into the bloodstream, and carbon dioxide moves in the opposite direction. The human lung is incredibly efficient at this – its sponge-like structure has the same surface area as a tennis court. The blood then moves into larger and larger branches until it is returned to the heart. A problem with either airflow or blood flow in the lung circuit will prevent gas exchange.

"So, parts of the lung get different amounts of air, ventilation, and different amounts of blood flow, depending on gravity and the position of the patient. When the patient is upright, the lung ventilates easily, but the blood flow is very dependent on gravity, with most of the blood flow going to the bottom of the lungs. This means that there are large parts of the lung with lots of air, but no blood, and the bottom of the lung has more blood than air. This is a mismatch." Dr Desmond draws another lung, horizontally, facing down. "Now, this is a patient on their front, in the prone position. The blood now flows to the lowest point, but that is a larger area of lung, and matches better with the lung being ventilated, meaning gas exchange is improved. There are a few other things that make it easier, but that's the nub of it."

No one, even Dr Desmond, seems sure why proning is so effective in COVID pneumonia patients, but we do know that for some patients, it's the only thing that makes a significant difference,* so we get a team together to "prone" Ali. As you can imagine, turning a human being, hooked up by five or more

---

* https://www.thelancet.com/journals/lanres/article/PIIS2213-2600(20)
30268-X/fulltext

different lines, including a life-saving breathing tube and medicine infusions, a human that is paralyzed and asleep, with no muscle tone, weighing sometimes well over 100 kg, is not a simple process. A lot can go wrong, including misplacing the breathing tube, dislodging lines, causing trauma to the bladder catheter and causing pressure damage to the face, eyes or ears. We assemble six people plus one person – Dr Desmond – who is "airway" trained, and we begin a complicated waltz through a checklist of strict actions, making sure everyone knows who is doing what when, ensuring we have the right drugs and that all the emergency equipment is readily available and working. Then we are ready to turn.

We line up, three on each side, with a special sliding sheet below Ali and three pillows placed on top of him. We then wrap a second bedsheet over the top, effectively cocooning him. Lastly, we protect Ali's eyes with soft gauze covers. Dr Desmond holds the airway tube and gives the directions. Pausing the ventilator means Ali is without air for a short time, so we need to be quick and efficient.

"On my count, halfway. One, two, three…" Dr Desmond instructs us.

We roll Ali halfway, held in mid-air on his side, tilted 90 degrees to the bed.

"Okay, change over," he says.

The two teams swap arms, from under the patient to over and vice versa.

"On my count, roll again, one, two, three…"

We roll Ali onto his front, gently placing his head and the breathing tube to one side, with the pillows now secure beneath him. We stretch one of his arms forward in what we call the "swimmer's" position, frozen mid-front-crawl. We restart the monitoring devices and the ventilator and run through the checks again. It all looks good. We let things settle, and then, over time, slowly try to reduce the ventilator settings. The oxygen comes down over a few hours, way past its previous level, and the blood gases continue to get better and better. We will have to turn him back over in 18 hours or so, which is referred to as "deproning", and see how he goes. But for now, at least, he's slowly receding from the edge.

We finish up the ward round, and then split up for breaks. After spending more than four hours in the PPE, I'm desperate to escape. I'm also very drained, having had nothing to eat or drink, not even water, and I'm finding the mask quite itchy, even irritative, especially to my eyes. I wonder if I'm mildly allergic. The headband of the visor squeezes around my temples and causes a headache that feels like a migraine – I make a mental note to mention to Nate to modify the design a little, to widen the band where it touches the head and relieve that pressure. Wearing two pairs of gloves starts making my hands itch, and I'm already scratching like crazy. Despite all this, I'm reluctant to leave the unit just yet, as longer stretches preserve the protective equipment, and we are currently binning equipment that is reusable, or could be reusable, in the midst of a global shortage. It seems mad. But my rumbling stomach and bleary eyes win out, and I go off to change and have a rest.

We have a specific room now, like an airlock between the "dirty" ward and "clean" areas. Doffing after several hours is a sweet relief. I'd got sort of used to the discomfort, but as a face-toucher, the freedom to rub my beard and eyes and feel normal again is bliss. I've let my beard grow back a little – there didn't seem much point shaving again given that the masks that I passed the fit-test with I've never actually seen again. Also, there was the prospect of a clean-shaven me being shunned by Dilsan and the kids again.

The mask, goggles and hair tie leave a criss-cross of lines and marks on my face. The first stop off is to the toilet, and then to hydrate. Lizzie comes down too. I've already got more used to seeing the other staff behind their visors and masks, and seeing their full faces again in the rest area is actually weird, and they're all similarly embossed with the marks left by hours of wearing masks and ties. I grab some food and there is free filter coffee and water, which I drink down greedily. I check my phone – the charity stuff is going really well, as Rosh's contact has just donated £50,000. It seems that people are really trying to get behind us.

I read a Sky News article that someone has posted in one of our WhatsApp charity groups about the Nightingale Hospital officially opening today. I didn't realize it's the world's largest critical care unit. It's an incredible undertaking, if not a little terrifying to think we will need 4,000 beds and possibly so much morgue space as well. I hope they start transferring some patients from here soon. Quite a few very senior and very good doctors I know on my social feeds seem to be involved, and I wonder how Hugo is getting on over there. It seems like they are starting small, so presumably he'll get phased in over the next few weeks with the other staff, staff from all around London and being shipped down from up north. I'm hopeful this might be the cavalry London needs. My hope is short-lived, however, because Nate forwards me a message from his manufacturer network. The Nightingale is looking for PPE stocks already, asking for local 3D-printed initiatives. The thought strikes me irritably that all of this was so avoidable.

What does give me a little confidence is that my social media and WhatsApp groups are filled with clinical discussions. Doctors from all over the country, including Italy, are connecting to share their on-the-ground experience as the situation develops. In many ways, the NHS is uniquely positioned to be great at this, with a national, highly motivated workforce. A summary lands in my inbox of the most recent national discussion on COVID care – already so much of the advice is changing. A picture is emerging of something different, a lung disease with local microscopic blood clots causing a great deal of the problems with lungs and kidneys. It's an impressively comprehensive and practical summary and finishes with a simple message: "Good luck, stay safe and be kind to one another." I take that message on board, as we don again and head back upstairs to the unit.

· · ·

We round the unit again in the afternoon, and Chloe and I come and check on Ali. He's doing much better on his front, the ventilator settings have been reduced and the blood gas analysis looks great. I don't recognize the nurse next to his bedside until she speaks. It's Dawn, one of the ward nurses from the cardiology ward. I forgot that they've all been drafted to become ICU nurses as well. It's her first day up here too, just like Chloe.

"How are you getting on?" I ask her.

"Oh, y'know. Made to move into intensive care… so…" The pause is filled with unspoken frustration and anxiety. I try to be reassuring.

"Me too. Have you worked in an ICU before?"

"No! I've been on the cardiac ward for 10 years."

I remembered that the nurses operate in siloed units, based on a specific ward, not just in a hospital. They form tiny families, working day in and day out, for years and even decades. Now they've been plucked from that familiar environment and thrust into this one, to fight a virus we are all really anxious about, without any of that support network they've had for years and years. For me, this jump has been a comparatively small one, but for Dawn, it's been a leap across an ocean. She is buddied with Kayla, an experienced ICU nurse who is showing her the ropes, but it's still a monumental change.

We are interrupted by the nurse beside her, as the patient next door is alarming. Not a patient I know well, I rush over, trying to rapidly assess the observations and the ventilator. The patient is a middle-aged but very frail-looking lady, coughing while connected to a breathing tube, an unusual situation caused by the ventilator getting confused and struggling to give breaths at the right time. Also, the oxygen saturation level looks like it's disappeared. For a moment I freeze, like I did all those years ago at the start of my training, staring at Florence, and attempting to deal with an emergency in unfamiliar territory. Just breathe, I think to myself. And then some distant cogs begin to spin, and I take a look at the monitor and see that the heart rate and blood pressure are fine. I do the few manoeuvres we've been taught and ask for suction. The nurse on this side passes me a suction catheter that isn't connected to anything, and I realize she is another of the training ward nurses, one I don't know. I manage to suction the tube correctly using the attached kit and pull the crash bell anyway in case I'm out of options. Thirty seconds later, half the team in two units is by the bedside, but the patient has stopped coughing, and it turns out that the saturations probe has just slipped off. No emergency. I'm a little embarrassed that she is completely fine, but Dr Desmond just shakes his head.

"That's exactly the right thing. Rush to wait, Dom, rush to wait," he tells me, reassuringly.

We've barely finished here when the bell goes off again – one of Lizzie's patients, John, a 56-year-old surveyor on day 7 of COVID pneumonia, is not doing very well in another bay. Lizzie hands him over to the crash team as we rush in. He had been doing okay, but all of a sudden, after moving his position to prevent bed sores, his oxygen level plummeted. As we are moving around him, it occurs to me that he's the same age and height as my uncle, with an Indian-sounding last name. The ward is entirely populated with BAME patients, people with brown or black skin, people who look like me, which backs up the general experience around London hospitals. And nearly all of them are men. Dr Desmond decides we should prone John as well, and tasks me to update his family.

It's slightly strange that I haven't spoken to a relative of a patient for quite some time in person, which would normally be a daily activity. Instead, we phone the next of kin. I dial the number awkwardly as I'm conscious that through the mask it isn't easy to speak that clearly. A lady named Sandra answers. It's a difficult conversation – expectations are so difficult to manage with COVID. Patients seem to deteriorate so rapidly, but we don't want to be overly pessimistic with relatives, even though some of the initial data from other intensive care units is very grim already. Equally, we can't be too optimistic either, and there's so much uncertainty around so much of what we are doing that it's hard to relay that with the confidence that a relative wants or needs, especially when they can't visit. I update Sandra about John's deterioration.

"I don't understand, he was fine this morning?" she says.

"He was stable, yes, but we are seeing this a lot. We are going to move him onto his front and see if that helps."

"Have you tried Vitamin C?" she enquires.

I'm not sure if I've misheard that. "What do you mean?" I ask.

"I've been doing a lot of reading – have you tried Vitamin C in a drip yet? What about… oh, what was it? Hold on." There's a rustle of paper before she says: "High-droxsy-chlorock-quin."

It takes me by surprise a little bit. Vitamin C drips have been touted as a possible treatment, although nowhere credible as yet, and hydroxychloroquine is an anti-malaria medication that may have some promise, although the reports are conflicting. In any case, we aren't using either of those routinely, and as far as I'm aware, nowhere is, outside of trials. I don't want to be dismissive toward Sandra; the advice is changing daily after all, and the next phone call she gets might be far worse news.

"Neither as yet – I think they're both quite experimental. I'll certainly ask about it, and we can let you know how it goes, moving him onto his front."

"Okay, thanks for the update."

I check for questions and then hang up, with a promise to call back later.

When I get back to John's room he is on his front already, proning complete. His numbers look marginally better. Satisfied, the team are starting to drift away.

Dr Desmond stops them.

"Not so fast, everyone, we need to prone bed 11 too."

And so we go on. It's hard physical work, proning patients, rushing back and forth as they dip and wobble, trying to get all the other jobs and phone calls done as well, and the routine ward rounds. Then the crash alarm goes off in the ICU next door, and we rush to help.

• • •

By handover time, I feel very strung-out. My eyes are itchy again and I feel fuzzy and distant, a low-level headache squeezing at my temples again. I must be dehydrated, probably something to do with not making it down for a second break. Chloe and I update the list and Lizzie helps us get down all the figures for the night team. We go through all of the stories again, sitting with the night team. It's pleasing to note that at least two patients, Ali and John, are doing much better than this morning, although so many others, like Deirdre, aren't. Lizzie and I are both exhausted, and I struggle to get through my patients in good time. Lizzie rolls her eyes and whips through hers succinctly like a pro. It's nearly 9 p.m. by the time we can finally leave the unit. Struggling out of the PPE again at the end is like peeling off a plaster, my skin raw and sensitive to the cool open air. I try to get down to get in the shower quickly, but find a queue already there.

On the drive home I call Dilsan and catch up – she is really energized. The food trucks we were trying to organize are now going ahead, our donation total has nearly reached £300,000, and the hospice that my friend was worried might have to close is staying open this weekend. With so much darkness in the world, Dilsan's voice is like a lighthouse, getting me home. I feel beaten up by the time I get there. Dilsan makes me strip and shower and I can barely make it through a conversation before collapsing into bed.

* * *

I wake up feeling like jelly, and much earlier than I'd like. I get ready quietly, and I'm in the car before 7 a.m. I think I only see a single car on the road for most of the journey into central London. Driving along the empty streets to park in deserted car parks is eerie. The hospital has made all coffee and food on site free, even at night. It's a huge relief to remember that when I realize I've missed breakfast at home again. The canteen fry-up isn't making the Michelin list any time soon but tastes like life itself. Even the filter coffee goes down like dark, liquid gold. I grab a muffin and chomp on it on the way to get changed. There are more staff in the rest area than I think I've ever seen gathered in one place in the hospital before – we are using it as a staging area for the two full intensive care units outside, and planning to cross-train staff today to open a third imminently. It strikes me as not the best idea, actually, to gather all together like this in a pandemic.

I bump into Lizzie again downstairs.

"How are you feeling?" I ask.

"Eurgh," is her reply, and it's a sentiment I share. "You?"

I laugh. "The same. I wonder if I'm mildly allergic to some of the kit, actually – my hands have come out in odd tiny raised bumps which are really itchy."

We head upstairs and hear about the progress of the patients overnight. There are several new ones, and we are struggling to add beds to take more. It's an incredible thing to be a part of, the Herculean effort across the board to meet the wave of the pandemic head-on and deal with it. It's a privilege to behold. But tensions are already running high, and we are all struggling to adjust to the new world, a world that seems to be swept from under our feet and replaced every day.

The night team have proned another patient, meaning we will have at least four patients today to deprone. Dr Desmond suggests we deploy "proning" teams, whose only job is to go patient to patient and flip them. Normally considered a last-ditch attempt to improve a severely unwell patient's oxygenation, Lizzie asks if there is an upper limit to the number of times we can prone-deprone somebody with COVID. Certainly, we wouldn't do it repeatedly for many other conditions, at least in adults.

Dr Desmond is ambivalent.

"We don't know. But if it works, we should do it. Lord knows, little else does," he says.

The early data we have from other countries suggests patients in intensive care are generally unlikely to recover after a long period on the ventilator, but equally, we are just about matching capacity as patients come flying in, marching through the hospital, taking over ward after ward, dragging staff and equipment behind us. Here at least, unlike some other units, we haven't come up against the hard wall of finite resources yet. The handover is accompanied by the inevitable whispers that follow the new incoming patients, from transfer teams and referral conversations, of what is going on in the wider world. We hear that a major hospital in north London has had to close, and several others have reached critical capacity, but this is typically downplayed in medic style as "having a tough time". That puts it somewhat mildly. We divide the ward again, and round our patients again. Ali is still on his front but doing much better. Chloe and I jot down a time to turn him back over later. Dawn seems more comfortable with things today, possibly because her patient is doing much better, but also thanks to the experience and confidence she's gained. Everyone is learning on the job, I suppose.

I'm relieved to find that John is much-improved. I volunteer to update Sandra at lunchtime – it would be good for her to get the same doctor on the phone two days in a row. We are making small gains, day by day, and that's the best we can hope for in an ICU like this. Our newest patient is a colleague, a radiographer, in his late fifties; originally from Wales, Kevin is well known to quite a few of the staff as "Kev". Dr Desmond knows him really well, and he's a familiar face to me to say hello to. Kevin fell ill only last week, working in areas thought to be "clean", but several patients had come through with coronavirus unknowingly, which was diagnosed on chest scans after the fact. Whether Kevin was exposed there, it's impossible to tell. He's now desperately unwell, with spiking temperatures, and his kidneys are teetering. His face is now warped, covered in lines and tubes and securing tapes, and slack in his unconsciousness.

Chloe is back with us, and as we round, we take particular care with Kevin's case, dotting and crossing every i and t. No more so than any other patient, I suppose, but everyone can't stand the idea of missing something with Kevin. It could be any of us on that bed in his place. We plan to start Kevin on kidney replacement if he doesn't improve, as his blood salts are yo-yoing up and down to dangerous levels. Kevin isn't our only healthcare professional – nearly a quarter of the ward patients across both ICUs have some sort of healthcare background; there are several doctors, mostly GPs, and some nurses. Too many healthcare workers are here. We make a note to return to put in some lines for Kevin's kidney machine in the afternoon.

The day is hard work. We need to flip back four patients, two of whom deteriorate within hours and need to be proned almost immediately back again, but John and Ali seem okay, for now at least. In between cases, I put the line into Kevin, which involves a slightly nerve-wracking 20 minutes trying to manipulate the ultrasound machine and avoid getting tangled between lines and tubes. All the while, I'm sweating and anxious about making a mistake, even in a simple procedure like this, I think just because he is a colleague. It all goes fine in the end, though.

The ward is jumpy. There don't appear to be enough nurses to keep opening beds, and other hospitals are calling incessantly, meaning that Dr Desmond is having to field phone calls in the middle of other tasks. It feels like all of London is starting to bear down on us. The nurses are as knackered as we are.

I help them cover their breaks by sitting with a few of the sickest patients while they are downstairs. I'm surprised at how grateful they are – clearly this isn't how the ward normally works. Dr Desmond puts it best when I mention nurses and doctors normally not crossing over like this: "We are all just one team now," he says.

In my break I flip through my phone again. Watford General has reportedly run out oxygen, and there are reports of a child of just five dying with coronavirus. Dilsan is really disturbed by that. She messages me to call her.

"I thought children weren't affected," she says.

"Not 'not affected', but just hardly any severe cases," I answer.

"Well, a child in the UK has died."

"Out of how many patients, though? In the community there could be a million cases by now, we are only testing a fraction of that. One in a million is too long odds to worry about. Better to worry about driving."

"I'm not driving, though," Dilsan quips, before sighing with frustration. "How is it there?"

"Busy. Getting busier. Nurses are overwhelmed."

"Can you not just come home?"

"Nearly there now, and then a few days off."

"It's not really 'off', though, is it?"

She has a good point – with our kids and the charity, our days are full to beyond bursting. We've little time for anything much else.

"This won't last forever," I say, trying to be reassuring.

"You don't know that."

"What do you mean?"

"I read a paper – I'll send it to you."

Dilsan sends me an article about coronavirus moving from a pandemic to becoming endemic, perpetually circulating around the world like influenza does, and the potential for different strains to arise in the future. It's frankly terrifying, and more than I can deal with right now. There's more than enough to be getting on with here, and I head back upstairs to finish the shift.

• • •

On the drive home, the day's patients swirl around in my head, as do Dilsan's concerns about the effects on children, and the possibility of a permanent twilight of COVID. Nej phones me on the in-car Bluetooth about some issues around the charity, and we get to chatting a bit more generally. The legal stuff, the financials, the constant pull to deliver more and more, to do more and more. It's exhausting. I'm still running on the buzz of energy that being released from work brings, but underneath, I'm bone-tired. Nej can hear it in my voice.

"Look, we aren't trying to solve everything here, there's a lot we just have to accept. We'll do what we can, and that's more than enough. Okay?"

"One foot in front of the other."

"Exactly. Let's catch up on Monday."

Nej rings off. I'm only 20 minutes from home, driving along at 25 mph up the high street. A glare off to the right makes me swerve slightly, and a blaring horn makes me correct rapidly, as a black sedan comes roaring past at what must be well over 70 mph. On nearly every trip I see some idiot doing the same, but it's the first time I've had a near-miss like this. I drive home very slowly, my knuckles white on the steering wheel. I tell Dilsan about it when I slump through the door. She looks really worried. A friend of hers works at one of the trauma hospitals, where she herself worked a few years back.

"They haven't seen a drop in car-accident trauma *at all*."

"That's incredible. There's hardly anyone out there."

"But the ones who are are driving like morons."

I resolve to get a cab the next day, as I fall asleep almost immediately.

· · ·

The next day, I do decide to get a cab. There's no traffic, it's a bright Sunday morning, and there are reams of emails and messages to catch up on with the charity, on top of going through my ICU notes app. It's quite relaxing in many ways – I try to use the free NHS uber discount, but it's already run out. I make a mental note to see if we can get a partnership sorted with the charity. I get to work early, knowing the route into the ICU now, so find myself sitting down to a free breakfast of sausage, beans and fresh hash brown, brown sauce and ketchup with a clear half hour of nothing to do before the shift starts.

I take a break from work/charity and catch up on my Scrabble games. I've started to play Scrabble with my mum, who's just got a phone that can finally have apps like Scrabble on it. We're quite competitive. It's a nice way to keep in touch. By the time it comes to get changed, I'm feeling very relaxed. Morale is actually quite cheap, I reflect – a little time, a little rest, some free food, all things we're focusing on with the charity. It's the last day of three here as well for our team, and everyone's spirits are lifted.

The handover blunts our mood somewhat, though. John has had to be proned again overnight and so has Ali. Kevin is worse, and there are plans to try to open a third ICU at the hospital within the next 24 hours to accommodate more patients. Dr Desmond is looking stressed. Several of his colleagues are isolating at home and every department is stretched; I feel like he's here all the time now. We split the ward round again. It's really quite strange to go round a ward where every patient has the same disease, a disease with very few treatment options. All we can do is do the small things well, support each patient through and try to scoop up the ones that fall down.

I join the proning team for the afternoon – we work across both ICUs at the hospital now. We deprone two patients and have to prone two more. It's physical work in full PPE. By the evening handover, it feels like we have gone the long way round to nowhere and everybody is back where we started. But equally, as the night registrar points out, everybody is still here. It's a very good point. A point we can take solace from, I suppose. It takes a long while to get changed, showered and finally outside waiting for a cab again. I get in and I try to do some work but fall asleep, waking outside my home, with the driver gently letting me know we are here. Slightly embarrassed, I stumble out and into the house. I don't think I've ever been this tired after a set of shifts. I'm dehydrated, and drained of every energy: physical, mental, moral.

Dilsan meets me at the door, takes my clothes and marches me up to the shower. The kids' bathwater is draining as I get in and feels cool against my feet while the hot water washes away a lot of the strains of the weekend. I get changed in the bedroom, sitting on the edge of the bed. I lie down for just a second. Dilsan finds me dead to the world and tucks me in. We haven't had a chance to say two words to each other. I sleep till lunchtime the next day.

. . .

I emerge feeling run-down, but happy to be home. Dilsan brings me a cup of tea and slides her phone alongside it.

"Johnson is in ICU," she says.

I'd completely missed the news that the Prime Minister, Boris Johnson, had been hospitalized somewhere yesterday, but I didn't find it particularly surprising. If he was going to deteriorate, then now would be the time, roughly a week after becoming symptomatic. And regardless of whether he needed a ventilator or not, he would be a very high-profile patient. Patients like him are often moved to intensive care, so as to keep them out of the public ward and get them into a secure part of the hospital. The last thing any hospital COVID ward needs is press and paparazzi.

He certainly isn't low-risk; he's in his late fifties and overweight. I don't know what will happen to him, or indeed who is running the country now at such a critical time. I figure that at least the lockdown message will perhaps sink in more widely now, though.

Despite being knackered, there is still too much to do on the charity front. Between the five of us trustees, we chair about 15 meetings over the course of the day, on potential partnerships with Spotify, website builds, legal, strategy – the list is endless.

There is some really positive news today, with Dilsan negotiating our first major partnership, with Percy's biscuit company. Juggling the kids and everything else is becoming really difficult. Unchecked, the calls alone could consume every day, and every one is so vital it's so hard to stop. Zach gets passed around the household, and Ayla is already asking me when all my "calls will be over". She likes to join some of them, but that seems to be par for the course in this new remote landscape that everyone is occupying during lockdown, with other people's kids, spouses and pets making regular appearances as well. It's nice, in a way – it feels like we're all in this together. I'm trying to give Dilsan a break – when I'm at work, she's on it full-time with the kids as well as all the charity work, and when I'm at home, I've got one toe in with the family and work nearly full-time on the charity as well. It's not enough. Being trapped in the house makes all of this 10 times as hard.

Dilsan has already explained to Ayla about the "germs" in my absence, so I'm slightly taken aback when Ayla asks if she can see her cousins "when the germs are over?" It's been hard to gauge what impact all this is having on the family, but this makes me feel like we haven't got it quite right. Dilsan and I separate the day a little bit, block off calls, and try to organize things better so we can manage it all. We draw a schedule on the cupboard.

Around lunchtime I flick through Twitter. An account called NursingNotes is tracking every healthcare worker death and has just posted about another nurse passing away. At least six doctors have also died by now that we know about. I show Dilsan. She suggests we set up a legacy project to create a lifelong cohort programme for education, opportunity and basic necessities for dependent children. It's a great idea.

"That sounds like a good idea, my love," I say.

Dilsan gives my hand a squeeze and gets on with the mountain of work we have to do.

Then I see an infuriating story on the *Telegraph Online*. "The inflexibility of our lumbering NHS is why the country had to shut down", reads the ignominious headline. I've literally never seen the NHS move so fast – we've tripled our ICU and kept going, and staff from all corners have jumped two-feet first into a crisis and just got on. I Tweet as much, but I wonder whether this headline is just clickbait trash, or whether there is a genuine crack in support for the NHS.

Nate messages me in the late afternoon. The printers have landed, and the farm is ready to set up.

"You coming down?" he asks.

I will need to pick up some of the visors and test them out before we can start thinking about supplying them. Too tired today, I defer to tomorrow. I switch off my phone in the afternoon – it really is endless. The kids need a bath and to get to bed, and I need to make some time for them. Disconnected from my phone, bath-time is a simple joy. Zach finds Ayla hilarious now, and they have started playing games, and even splashing each other. It's a mess and I love it. It's the small moments that keep me grounded. The kids don't care about 3D printers, PPE shortages, Boris Johnson in ICU – none of that exists for them. All that's important to them is their home and their family. It provides me with much-needed perspective – I need to remember that too.

That night is Nesli and Ehsan's anniversary, so we order separate takeaways and sit and chat over Zoom. Huddled around the laptop on the sofa, with a glass of wine, chatting and laughing, it's not like it was, but it's closer than we've been for a long time.

"We miss you guys," Nesli tells us.

"We miss you too."

"Do you think it'll ever be normal again?" Nesli asks.

Dilsan and I share a look. It'll be months as a minimum.

"There'll be a new normal, I guess," I say.

"We can get one of those special social distance hugging sheets maybe," Ehsan jokes, referencing a news report about a plasterer who designed a "cuddle curtain", comprising a transparent plastic sheet with sleeves to ensure that two people do not come into direct contact while hugging.

"I'm sure they are all sold out. Maybe we can make some at the print farm."

We all laugh.

When we ring off the quiet seems a little more obvious in comparison. Dilsan and I both really feel their absence.

. . .

The next morning, I find myself driving down deserted streets through central London, heading to the print farm at Somerset House on the bank of the Thames. As I park the car, I take a moment to marvel at the view – there is no one around. On the other side of the river, the National Theatre stands empty, as it has done for weeks. It's a blisteringly bright April day. It occurs to me that this is the first time I've been anywhere that wasn't work or home for a month. It feels good. The air near the water even smells clean, and I wonder if it's because there's so little traffic on the roads of London. I've seen photos of the waters in Venice, crystal clear, and wonder if something similar must be happening here.

Nate meets me at the entrance to Somerset House – we are careful to socially distance, which feels weird and socially awkward. He's his same laid-back self, but he's clearly excited. He gives me the tour of Somerset House as we descend into its bowels.

"This is where the old naval areas used to be, but some had to be rebuilt after the Blitz." His soft Californian accent echoes a little as we wander into the warren of new and old, spliced together. We eventually come out of these catacombs to a bright neon sign declaring this part of the building "Makerversity". Inside is a wide-open workshop, where row upon row of simple worktables has been set up. In the back room, 30 or so 3D printers are quietly humming away, the soft circular back and forth motion of their glass plates reminding me of swilling a fine glass of whisky. The printers themselves are, from the outside, basically simple black square boxes, but to see the farm, an idea only a week ago, in its infant reality is incredibly moving. Nate is buzzing – for him, this is years of theory suddenly in practice. It has also involved a tremendous amount of work, and many of the other Makerversity members are helping unload the boxes to get more printers set up. It suddenly dawns on me what a huge undertaking this will be. I record some footage to add to the SHIELD launch video and beam it back to the group – they are hugely impressed. It really is a magnificent sight.

I head back in the afternoon, parched and hungry, having foolishly forgotten to bring anything edible with me, loaded up instead with a selection of visors, respirators and even an experimental snorkel mask to test out. I give them a good clean when I get home – Dilsan makes me decontaminate as well. It's becoming a strange ritual. We do all the shopping whenever we get any as well, sitting on the hallway floor washing down everything wipeable. It seems like overkill sometimes, and then wholly needed other times. As new data crops up in the literature, my opinion ping-pongs back and forth.

We play with the kit on the kitchen table, assembling the visor and fit-testing the respirator. I try to mould it to my face by warming it in near-boiling water, but all I end up doing is nearly burning myself. I sit looking at all of this assorted ingenuity and marvel at the kindness and skill of the team at Makerversity.

· · ·

I'm back in the ICU from the end of the week, mercifully scheduled on the rota for a run of short days, though, which means I can get home in time, at a push, to see the kids. Time in the hospital has bounced forward again, like a stone skipping on a pond, and we have gone from two ICUs, to three, with a planned fourth one opening soon. Dr Desmond is still here, and I wonder if he's taken a break at all in the last week. Rumours abound about colleagues at home with COVID. I find my own 3D printed visor safe and sound on the unit, its rigid familiarity becoming something of a talisman on these shifts.

Many of the longer-term stable patients have been moved into other units, leaving only the sickest patients here, including two whose lungs are in such bad shape that they have been put on a super-advanced therapy called extracorporeal membrane oxygenation. ECMO is the last-ditch way of getting oxygen into the blood, which involves extracting the blood into a labyrinthine device that looks like something between an airplane engine and a coffee machine, before two huge tubes pass blood that has been artificially filled with oxygen back into the body. These can support the lungs (or the heart or both), and require super-specialist training to handle safely.

We start the day with a bang, literally, as the crash alarm to one of the side rooms goes off. Khalid is a 40-year-old optician, newly transferred last night after being "scooped" up from another hospital, his lungs more solid tissue than their normal aerated consistency, and looking more like the liver than a lung, a phenomenon we call hepatization. Essentially now inert blocks of flesh, the lungs barely move, and no air can get in to reach the bloodstream. The ICU team here went over to the hospital Khalid was in and put in all the very large-bore tubes to get him started on ECMO, bringing him back still attached to the machine. Even here, at the maximum level of life-support, Khalid is struggling.

The crash alarm has gone off because the ECMO machine is alarming, appearing to stutter and start. The flow has become interrupted and Khalid's saturations, the level of oxygen in the blood, is drifting slowly down and down, from 90 to 80 to 70. Another consultant, Dr Specter, is looking pensively at the ECMO machine, purposefully turning down the flow dial and bringing it up again, bit by bit. The alarms stop as Khalid's saturations start to drift back up again, his blood oxygen normalizing.

Dr Specter seems pleased, and she and Dr Desmond discuss what to do next with Khalid. The final opinion is to give him time, so that's what we do. One of the senior intensive care registrars does an ultrasound of Khalid's lungs that day – the diaphragm, the muscle that controls respiration at the bottom of the lungs, quivers pathetically against the weight of the congested lungs above. When we stop the ventilator for a tubing circuit change, Khalid's oxygen levels don't change at all. He is entirely dependent on the ECMO machine now.

Our next patient is Deirdre again. Deirdre has been on the unit for three weeks now, initially very up and down, but over the past few days she's entered a steady decline going only one way. The wrong way. She has slid steadily into needing more and more pressure to ventilate, and is already well above the maximum pressures we can safely deliver, her carbon dioxide levels in the blood increasing every single day. Her body is trying to adjust, and the numbers on her analysis are like none I've ever seen. When we go round, her latest blood gas figure is much worse again, showing a carbon dioxide level we can do little to improve, and increasingly acidic blood. Her kidneys have shut down, and a machine to replace them ticks and whirs quietly by her bedside. The chest X-ray paints an even grimmer picture, showing two masses of knotted scar tissue, almost totally white where the clear black spaces of a chest film should be. Her lungs are slowly petrifying, and her other organs are failing as well.

We go through the motions on the ward round, examining her from top to tail, looking through her charts, her medicines. She's had a round of steroids, another treatment we have been trying in a speculative fashion based on some of the case reports from elsewhere, but without much benefit. There's little to add here. Dr Desmond recognizes that long before I do. Deirdre's lungs are terminally failing, she is dying, and is too frail to survive going on to something like ECMO, even if we had the resources to offer it to everyone.

"Should we call the family?" I ask.

"I think so," Dr Desmond answers, looking bleak.

We are still not allowing visitors onto the unit, for infection control reasons as much as for the impracticality of shuttling members of the public in full PPE in and out of intensive care rooms on a regular basis. We have adaptations, updating a regular point of contact on the phone and now even facilitating video calls. But at the very end of life, where we think Deirdre is now, we allow family members and religious counsel to come in to say their final goodbyes. I give her son, Mark, a call through the muffled mask of full PPE.

"Hello?" Mark's voice is deep, slightly cracked. The strain of having a relative on ICU with coronavirus must be unimaginable, especially with all the wall-to-wall media coverage.

"Hello. I'm Dom, one the doctors looking after your mum."

"Oh. Hullo." From what I can gather from the notes, this is a call Mark has been expecting for some time. I explain Deirdre's continuously failing lungs, the very high pressures we are already on, the worsening blood gases. We have nowhere to go.

"Should I come in, then?" Mark asks.

It's always a difficult question. I've called plenty of family members in to see their dying relatives for their final goodbyes, only to be proven wrong, even eventually discharging one patient home. We can never really give timeframes, so I just go with what I would want if it was my mum.

"I think that would be a good idea, Mark."

"Okay." He hangs up the phone very quietly.

The ward sister in charge a few hours later ushers Mark onto the ward, awkwardly tall in full PPE, into the bay to sit at his mother's bedside and hold her hand. It's the first visitor she's had in nearly a month. And will be, I'm sorry to say, her last. Her blood has become too acidic, having a domino effect across all of her body functions, organ after organ failing as well. There's nothing to reverse. We switch off the observations and the blaring alarms, and as the bay fills with the mid-morning sun, it's quiet at the bedside. Mark holds her hand, only his grey-blue eyes visible above the mask. I give him some space and see to another patient. Dr Desmond talks to Mark for some time, and sits beside him as the machines are finally switched off. She passes away peacefully minutes later. Despite the strange times, the environment, the lockdown, Deirdre has a humane and dignified death, with her family beside her. It's the best we can give.

* * *

Ali is still on the ward, already holding the record for being proned and deproned again more times than any other patient. The odds are increasingly stacked against him – he's going on to a kidney replacement machine, he has a new chest infection and he's on high-dose antibiotics, while the nurses struggle to keep his blood thin enough for the kidney machine but thick enough to stop him bleeding from lines and his breathing tube.

He's been on a ventilator for nearly a month at this point – and every day the update to the family is the same: "Stable, but remains critically unwell". I can't imagine the agony of a loved one dangling at this point for a day, let alone weeks. Despite the fluctuations, he's managed to stay a few days without needing to be proned again, although he remains on very high ventilator settings. We don't make any changes, and move on. There's this constant tension, as if what we are doing here is futile, while the pace and flow of patients suggests many many more will soon need these beds. And yet, we persist. No one seems convinced there is a right answer.

"Hopefully the Nightingale will take some of these patients?" I ask, seeing as the hospital is now open, although I had heard they had only taken 20 or so patients to date.

Dr Desmond shrugs before saying:

"It's quite a narrow criteria to get over there – you need to have only one organ failing at the moment, and all of ours here have at least two. One patient was referred to the Nightingale Hospital but got sent back, which is a total waste of resources." Then his phone rings for what must be the hundredth time that morning and he strides away. I make a mental note to message Hugo – now working at the Nightingale – to hopefully shed some light on it when I can reach my phone, which is currently wrapped in a blood specimen bag in my scrub pocket beneath the gown.

The ebb and flow of ICU, especially COVID-ICU, is long periods of inactivity, broken up by often dire emergencies. There are only so many parameters to manage, only so many levels of escalation to go through, and fundamentally, what the patients need is support and time and careful vigilance against other infections. We do our morning ward rounds, arrange our breaks, divide the jobs, if there are any, and react to any deteriorating or new patients. We do the afternoon round, arrange our breaks, type up the long list of parameters for the handover, and go home. Rinse, repeat.

On my way out for the lunch break I notice that we have started to reuse the goggles and visors, which makes sense, dunking them in big buckets of cleaning fluid and then in water before letting them dry. Given the size of our ICUs now, I imagine that must be someone's full-time job every day. I wonder if perhaps we should start exploring reusing everything. I check my phone – the charity group is abuzz with the news that we have just blown past £500,000 in donations, as the new campaign with the Maddox Gallery seems to be hitting the stratosphere already. Nate pings me some videos of the first batch of visors being printed, over a thousand of them, humming away in the farm.

I get some lunch and wander back for some quiet time in the new "relaxation room". The Trust has been slowly building rest and relaxation facilities, a kitchen, a TV room, and now a relaxation room, cannibalizing clinic rooms that are currently lying fallow. The relaxation room includes four comfy chairs, a surprisingly tasteful lamp and a coffee table, apparently donated by Made.com, the furniture company. Someone's left a copy of *The Boy, The Mole, The Fox and The Horse* by Charlie Mackesy. I've never picked it up before, and I flick through the pages. "If at first you don't succeed," it reads, in a curled script almost like calligraphy, "have some cake."

I snort out loud. As a motto for the NHS, I couldn't think of a better one. What a strange and thoughtful book to leave in this particular room, I think to myself. Despite my initial scepticism, I do start to feel a lot more relaxed after a very difficult morning.

Dilsan messages me while I'm there.

"How's work?"

"Bit rough. How's home?"

"Bit rough."

"Not too long now, home early tonight!"

Although by the time we hand over and I change, shower and start the drive back, it's already nearly 7 p.m. When I creep in, both the kids are asleep. I vow to try and exit more promptly tomorrow.

• • •

The next day we are combing through the patients once more – Ali and Kevin are thankfully no worse, but no better either. Kevin has been started on a course of steroids in the hope it might shift things in the right direction, although there's not much guidance for that. Dr Desmond is discussing what we should do with steroids when the emergency buzzer interrupts us, on the ICU next door. We rush over there and I recognize the patient beneath the hands of the emergency team. It's John again, his oxygen suddenly critically low. Another registrar I don't know detaches the ventilator and attaches a manual airbag to the tube, gently squeezing air into John's lungs with one hand (a technique known as "bagging"). The registrar looks up when Dr Desmond arrives.

"Looks like he's plugged off," he says, gesturing to a small wad of thick, dry secretions in the suction catheter.

The emergencies have started to worry me – not so much for myself, but for my senior colleagues, especially the anaesthetists. The airway emergencies I can only really pull the buzzer for and press the oxygen button on the ventilator (the only time I'm touching the ventilator), but I watch as more senior colleagues perform emergency procedures, changing tubes and "bagging" – all procedures which produce the most infectious particles, aerosols, in very high numbers. In normal circumstances, this is the right thing to do in an emergency, but with the COVID patients, it seems like we should be doing as little of this type of work as possible, an opinion that at least one of the bosses shares. Paranoid about this, I hand Dr Desmond my visor to swap for his goggles and chivvy the other unneeded staff out of the room. Several of the ICU consultants have become sick already, one seriously so.

The physiotherapist arrives to help do some manoeuvres to clear the blockage, rhythmically tapping the chest and rolling the patient to loosen up and suction away the problem. Quickly, John's levels return to normal. It's a process that exposes everyone nearby to aerosols, and I anxiously check the seal on my mask just in case. We debate whether proning again might help, but decide to watch and wait.

The NHS machine is in full motion now, in fifth gear and running smoothly, oiled with the titanic efforts of my colleagues. As we are charging forward to keep pace with the pandemic, we have to cancel all work other than the life-or-death emergencies. Like the water building behind a dam, all of those appointments, cancer surgeries, heart surgeries, are piling up in the community. We were already sitting on the worst healthcare waiting lists since records began, long before the pandemic started, and now I dread to think how we will cope nationally after this. And it's not just the planned patients we will have to eventually deal with – it will be all the unplanned, non-COVID patients that seem to have vanished, or, worse, are delaying coming into hospital when they need to. Anecdotally, at least, we are seeing more delayed heart attacks and their complications: damaged heart tissue leading to ruptures and flailing, dysfunctional heart valves, which are often deadly.

During my break, I wander over to the new units, the cardiac ward I used to work on. I recognize the same geographical landmarks as before the pandemic, but these are COVID wards now, and everything feels like it's in an alternate dimension. Everyone is in PPE, and no one brings anything to or removes anything from the ward. Every ward bed, so recently populated with a cardiology patient, is now occupied by a COVID patient on a ventilator. Where are all the patients that were once here? The thought chills me, as I think of what we will be facing when all this is over.

. . .

My itchy hands have now progressed to becoming permanently inflamed, thickened, red and crusty. The skin occasionally breaks, so when I use the hand sanitizer, the alcohol stings. During the long shifts I keep forgetting and automatically sanitizing them when I doff, duly reminded again as they burn with the gel. It's incredibly frustrating. I keep meaning to get to the pharmacy to pick up some sort of topical treatment but can never seem to find the time. When I get home that night, Dilsan tsks to see how bad they've become. I ping a photo of them over to a friend of mine, Christina, from medical school, who has just become a dermatology consultant. It seems completely unbelievable to me to imagine we were only students together 10 years ago.

"Whose hands are those?" she asks, thinking this is one of my referrals.

"They're mine!" I reply.

"Oh God," she answers. Hmmm – not the best reaction. "Can you take one with your ring off?" she asks.

I remove my wedding ring to expose the white but otherwise unblemished skin and take another photo.

"Looks like a contact allergy." She gives me a long list of creams and instructions. I'm incredibly grateful I can just call up a colleague to help with this. How many of these types of problems are getting ignored in the community right now, I wonder.

Beck looks over my shoulder.

"Eurgh," she says, grinning.

"Thanks, Beck."

"You should try this," she says, pulling some organic oat cream (or similar) from her potions box, which happens to be next to her. I dab a few spots on and find that it gives quite good relief.

"See, I should be a doctor," she says, laughing.

Living with Beck is going really well – it's a big change in our home dynamic, but a positive one. She's a great roommate –

she tidies, cooks and even mows the lawn. Not to mention her seemingly bottomless list of connections for the charity. Most importantly, the kids adore her, especially Zach, who considers her his favourite person in his pantheon of grown-ups. Despite that, the charity has put an occasional strain on our relationship – wearing too many hats between us gets confusing and causes things to become easily heated. She puts it down to "growing pains" and we resolve our differences.

On Monday 13 April, I catch up with my mum, partly to gloat over winning our recent online Scrabble games, but also to see how she is doing. Not only is she shepherding Dad through lockdown, she also has to keep my gran (living alone with mild dementia) going too. Organizing carers and home support is difficult at the best of times, let alone during lockdown. We give her a call on FaceTime. Ayla sits and eats her dinner and tells her about her day.

"How's Gran?" I interject, interrupting a fictitious story about one of Ayla's many imaginary sisters (she has at least a dozen now, and we've started thinking that she's trying to hint something to us).

"Oh, not too bad. Getting a bit more vague about details, I suppose. We are managing."

"And Dad?"

"Well, he has now been convinced that staying at home doesn't include Waitrose, so I think he's alright."

It occurs to me that we haven't seen each other in person since January. Zach has grown up so much now. That must be really hard for Mum, who lives for her grandchildren.

"And how are you, Mum?"

"You know, not too bad. We are working from home now, so that's okay. Just getting on with it, really."

Mum is being quite stoical, but I sense that this is a particularly hard time for her.

"Let's try and have some regular calls?" I suggest. "We can start with bedtime?"

That night I pop Grandma on FaceTime and she reads a bedtime story to Ayla from my screen perched on Ayla's doll's house. Ayla loves it. It makes a big difference.

∙ ∙ ∙

Over the week the charity grows and grows, edging unbelievably closer to the £1 million mark in donations. Nej whips the organization into shape, expanding it with a network of skilled and dedicated volunteers. Our SHIELD initiative picks up some press attention and "BBC Breakfast" interviews me about our work and the charity, and asks what it has been like leaping from cardiology to the ICU. It's a question I've not really prepared for, so I answer honestly; for us it's a small hop, but it's the nurses that have had to leap a chasm and they don't get nearly enough praise for it, especially in the media.

The pressure to deliver the visors is on now. The "farm" at the Makerversity at Somerset House is being run by Nate and Tim Burrell-Saward, one of the other Makerversity members running multiple PPE projects, but they aren't manufacturers. They're having to learn on the job what material is needed, and when it is needed by. We have 400 visors due for urgent next day delivery by Paul and contractors appeal to a medical centre in Stockport, and I message Nate to find out if we can get this out on time. He's been pulling all-nighters getting the place set up for a week now.

"Yeah, should be fine, I'll keep you posted," he messages me at 5 p.m.

Slightly concerned by the time, but hopeful, I put the kids to bed and sit down with Dilsan to do some work on the charity. I message Paul again at 7 p.m.

"How's it looking?"

"Might need a few more hours, if I'm honest," Paul replies.

This means that we will miss the slot for delivery, with maybe a delay of days to get another.

I phone Paul.

"We can pick it up from your house first thing tomorrow, on the drive up to Stockport?"

There isn't really much choice, if we want to get it out as soon as possible. I text Nate.

"Okay, I'm coming down to help."

* * *

After mainlining a couple of coffees to wake myself up again, I find myself back in the car around 9.30 p.m., driving down deserted central London avenues, dotted with empty orange pools of lamplight. Despite the lack of other cars, I drive slowly and deliberately, acutely aware that a reckless driver could pop up at any moment. It makes for a reflective, even peaceful, journey. The streets truly are empty, including of the homeless, who have been sheltered in hotels around the capital. One of the few good things about this crisis is that homelessness has ended, even if just for a little while. It's also essentially happened overnight. It's incredible to think how quickly things can be achieved once the desire and energy are there.

I pull up outside Somerset House – it's a warm night and the Thames flows steadily alongside. The air smells fresh. Suddenly invigorated by the freedom, despite the late hour, I feel full of energy. Perhaps it's the two coffees kicking in, but when Nate greets me at the barrier, I am ready to work. Unfortunately, there is a lot of work to do; the laser cutter needs to be run another 50 or so times, and then each individual plastic sheet needs to be hand-washed before it's ready to be used as eyewear. So, for the next three hours, up to 2 a.m., I am doing the washing up. The glamorous life of a print farmer. We get 400 visors boxed and packaged and into my car, and then I drive home again, leaving the visors, ready to go out in just a few hours, on our doorstep. I make a mental note, as the manic energy dissipates as my head hits the pillow, to sort out a project manager for this kind of stuff in future so I don't need to do that again.

* * *

It's been an exhausting week all round, and by the time I come back to the hospital for a set of night shifts on Friday, I'm already bone-tired. The charity donors are also keen for an update, so I find myself waiting for an Uber, sitting on my garden wall, chatting on a conference call to Joe Cole about 3D-printed visors and celebrity chef food drops. I used to collect Panini stickers for my football albums with his face on. It's such a strange moment, going down one rabbit hole in ICU and another with the charity at the same time. I've spoken to a few of my colleagues – this feeling of surreality, of un-reality, isn't unique.

A combination of trauma, increasingly strange and frightening circumstances, and that need to rise ever higher to keep one's head figuratively above water, means we are becoming more and more disconnected from the world we knew before. Once I'm off the phone I have a few moments in the back of the car to watch the world go quietly by, draped in the gold and auburn of the dying afternoon sun.

The hospital has taken another step deeper – we have six intensive care units now in total, with a plan to open two more if needed, and it's a struggle to work out where all the staff need to be going at each handover, so we have started gathering downstairs first, in the relaxation room, to work out who needs to cover where for the night. We sit around in full PPE, waiting for the handover. I notice that one member of the team I don't recognize is reading the copy of *The Boy, The Mole, The Fox and the Horse* – it's a really weird sight, seeing someone flicking through the pages of a book with gloved hands and peering over an FFP3 mask.

The team tonight for our unit are all very welcome interlopers, like I was, all seconded from other specialties. The consultant is a cardiology colleague and a friend, Dr Lam, and our junior is one of the respiratory doctors, although nearly a registrar himself, Athanasis. None of us being intensive care specialists, a further consultant, Professor Frith, will be rounding with us, covering several of the units up here fighting fires for the teams as they go. The consultants are always very stretched.

We step onto the cardiac ward, now converted into a full-size intensive care unit. It's completely different to how it would normally be, except for one key parameter, the temperature. Intensive care wards are usually significantly cooler than the general wards, but here, it's sweltering. The PPE is deeply uncomfortable. No one knows how to turn the temperature down – in these modern buildings, the air conditioning is a wild beast beholden only to itself. We've actually had to cancel procedures in the past when the temperature ran blazingly and inexplicably hot in the cath lab (the operating theatre-like areas in which cardiology procedures are performed). Apparently, the estates department, which usually deals with such things, has been contacted, which may or may not mean anything at all, given that it's the weekend. My mouth feels dry and my hands are on fire already, itching like crazy. I try to concentrate as I listen to the day team handover.

It sounds like it's been a busy day – patients are moving all around the hospital as we try to categorize them into levels of need. This area is becoming the "chronic" COVID unit, for patients who have mostly been here for longer than a month already. Many of them have been intubated and ventilated, and more than a few have had tracheostomies, the special tube inserted directly into their neck, so they're awake and breathing but still on the ventilator. Half the ward are on kidney replacement machines as well, which have proven to be particularly difficult to manage, with tiny blood clots frequently blocking the filter tubes, meaning we are burning through equipment twice a day for one patient with circuits that should last for a week. We are running out. And that's not the only thing. The drugs we use to sedate patients are in short supply worldwide, along with the drugs required for general anaesthetics. We've run through plan A, plan B, and are now stuck in plan C.

We've run out of the normal gowns as well, and white coveralls have appeared, made of the same material we shroud the dead in. They are also much more difficult to take off – they need to be stepped out of rather than stripped off, which is not how we have been trained to carefully remove the outer gown. I managed to find my own visor on the unit; the 3D-printed version has been sitting up here for four weeks now, and is still going strong. It's very rigid – I tap it twice with my pen for good luck and it makes a resounding and reassuring knock, knock sound as I do. Still my talisman. As we listen to a litany of grim stories, with very little hope in between, I tap it again more than once.

After the handover we go and see the patients, and I realize I've met several already, in what feel like past lives, years ago, not a few weeks prior. Professor Frith, who always seems to be on the move, joins us. In the corner of the unit is Maurice, a 71-year-old retired shopkeeper who has been on the unit for six weeks. He looks frail and drawn. Maurice has a past medical history a page long, from way before COVID came along. Intubated patients in ICU lose half their muscle mass within three days of being on a ventilator, and Maurice had little to begin with. He's been proned and deproned so much it takes Athanasis about a minute to count them up on the handover notes – 12 times. Each episode, Maurice wobbles, getting a little better, then a little worse, then a lot worse and here we are again. On the steep downward arm of another of those spirals, Maurice is struggling again. His blood has become acidic, which is making his blood pressure drop, the ventilator is struggling to keep his lungs going and we are needing to give more and more medicines to keep the blood pressure up. Professor Frith changes some of the ventilator settings but doesn't seem satisfied.

"Shall we get ready to prone?" I ask, standing between Dr Lam and the Professor, our eyes meeting through visors and over masks.

"Let me go and pow-wow with some of the other ICU consultants. Carry on the round, he's stable for the moment," Professor Frith says, before disappearing.

We continue on, pushing the computer on wheels to the next patient, Jeffrey, 58, who owns a pub and until recently was still working behind the bar. When I heard his occupation in the handover, I recalled all the media footage of packed bars and pubs immediately before the lockdown. I was angry about the crowds at the time, but never once gave a thought to those working there, with far less choice, far more exposed. Those like Jeffrey. He's been with us for over five weeks now, and had a tracheostomy tube placed last week at the base of his neck. He's now been woken up. But like so many older patients that have been under for so long, coming out and reorienting is an even longer way back. Jeffrey remains deeply confused, making very little eye contact, and he is unable to speak due to the tube, as air is diverted out through the tube before reaching the vocal cords, silencing them. It's a difficult balance – if Jeffrey becomes agitated he pulls dangerously at the lines and the ventilator tube, as well as the feeding tube into his nose, so we need to give some stabilizing sedation, but if he has too much, he is asleep again and no closer to recovery. Often, bringing family in can help, but we can't do that here either. For now, at least, Jeffrey seems comfortable, so there's little to do as the nurses follow the weaning process to reduce the ventilator. We keep going.

A patient I do know, Ali, is in the bed by the window. I look at the notes and see that they attempted a tracheostomy but it failed, causing air to track through the skin and into the chest, so a further tube was inserted into the chest before his lungs became compressed as well. Everyone up here has looked after Ali by now at some point. As we wheel the computer over, the nurse comes running to tell me "He's desaturating." Slightly perturbed from walking into an unheralded emergency, we crowd round the bedside as Ali's numbers slide down, requiring more and more oxygen to keep them level. I listen to his chest – it's crackly and quiet on both sides. Dr Lam makes a change to his ventilator settings and we order an urgent X-ray. In the middle of this, the crash alarm goes off; Athanasis stays with Ali and Dr Lam and I rush round to the end-bay, where the alarm's coming from. Professor Frith joins us as we reach the patient – it's the only other patient I know on the ward, Kevin, the radiographer and our colleague.

Kevin has gone from bad to worse over the weeks, requiring higher and higher pressures to ventilate. He's had a few stable days, but now appears to be not ventilating at all. The nurse is urgently suctioning mucous from this tube as the alarm blares, his oxygen levels sitting in the mid-60s (normal is between 94 and 100). Professor Frith studies the graphic of his breathing pattern – it seems to oscillate from a normal-looking one to a blunted one. A few more attempts to suction any blockages don't have any effect.

"Okay, we will need to re-intubate him," Professor Frith says. "Can you get the trolley, please?" He is calm, but his voice is strained. Professor Frith must be reaching retirement age, and intubating a COVID patient is one of the procedures that presents the highest exposure risk to the operator.

As we wheel the intubation trolley in, Dr Lam remembers that Ali still needs attention, on the far side of the ward.

Professor Frith doesn't bat an eyelid.

"Oh, it's probably the drain. Make sure it's on suction," he says. This means leaving the drain on negative pressure, to keep the air from accumulating in the chest. I rush back over to find Athanasis looking at the portable chest X-ray that's just been performed. There's a large, blank, black space where his right lung should be. Professor Frith was right. We check the drain, and sure enough, it isn't on suction. We open the tap and wait. Slowly, Ali's oxygen levels stabilize. Leaving Athanasis where he is, I return to Dr Lam and Professor Frith, who are about to change the tube for Kevin. They've cleared the bay to protect the other staff and I watch on from the door. They spend a lot of time preparing and then move very quickly, stopping the ventilator, removing the old tube and then inserting the instruments to pass the new tube in its place. Every second that passes is a second that Kevin isn't breathing. It's all the more gut-wrenching knowing that Kevin is a colleague, the closeness of his position to our own making everything more real. The seconds stretch and then snap back and he is connected to the ventilator again, breathing. The trace swings in a nice normal pattern. That's one fire put out.

We round back to Ali; with his chest drain working again, he is slowly righting, and the amount of oxygen he needs is coming down. We finish back where we started, with Maurice, still struggling despite the ventilator setting changes. His latest blood gas analysis is worse.

"What did you decide, Prof?" I ask.

"Hmm?"

"About proning?"

Professor Frith sighs.

"The decision was not to turn him again."

There's a pause. It's not unexpected, but it's still jarring to pivot away from an active treatment. We are accepting we can't make Maurice better, at least not enough to ever get off the ventilator. Continuing to endlessly flip him seems futile and cruel if that is the case.

Dr Lam pipes up.

"We should call in his family."

"That would be… wise," Professor Frith says.

The nurse makes the arrangements and we plan to speak to his niece when she arrives on the ward. It's already well past midnight as we finish the ward round. I'm parched, and it feels like the backs of my eyes ache with tiredness. Dr Lam sends me down for a break, and the ICU on-call registrar comes and relieves him. There's an ominous feeling as I'm going down in the lift. It feels like this weekend is going to be hard.

As the ICUs have expanded, with dozens more staff on each shift, so have the rest services. The pandemic is being recognized as a time of extreme unusual stress on the service, and the hospital and outside organizations, including our own charity, have stepped up the focus on staff wellbeing and rest facilities. The rest area evolves as the pandemic does, sprouting a kitchen and a TV area; the relaxation room continues to evolve, its latest offspring a small, square, coffee table. Periodically, treats or food arrive, and are consumed by the swarm of staff down here now, leaving the literal crumbs of digestive biscuits. All the food is free, and there is hot food available 24/7 from the cafeteria. Once considered a staple of working life in a hospital, this hearkens back to a bygone era of perks for hospital staff.

I wander along the corridor to find a queue, at 1 a.m., for hot food. To see so many people, even socially distanced, on a night shift is a heartwarming sight. Nights, especially for doctors who often work in very small teams or on their own, can be very lonely, especially without access to food and often even water. So it makes a wonderful change to bump into one of the junior docs I know well, Julie, and start chatting. The chef has just poured out a fresh batch of chips, and the smell curls into my nose and punches me in the uncus (the part of the brain that is stimulated by smell but also memory; I used to remember this in medical school by calling it the "odours and uncles" area). Sitting with a plate of steaming, crunchy fresh chips, dipped in ketchup, at 2 a.m., makes me reflect.

"How will we ever go back?" I ask Julie, gesturing with a chip.

"Back from what?"

"From this!" I again use a chip as a pointing device. "How did we ever do shifts without food at night? Alone and without rest areas? It seems criminally inhuman in comparison."

"Well, I presume after the pandemic we'll go back to normal?" This is typical of a 2 a.m. conversation – I think I'm waxing lyrical on the great problems of our time, and Julie thinks I'm talking bollocks.

I just shake my head.

"I think so much will change. It will have to – there'll be millions of patients on the waiting lists by the winter at this rate. We'll have to find some pretty novel ways of working. Telephone clinics are here to stay." I take another chip. "And when this is all over, on top of everything else, so many of us will just want a break. It'll be things like *this*," I say, pointing to my chips, "that keep people going."

"I guess." Julie shrugs, perhaps not as infatuated with chips as I am. I change the subject.

"Coffee?" I suggest.

I'm really starting to enjoy the free filter coffee. The percolating machine and the smell of a fresh jug is perhaps only beaten by the hot chips. The earliest documented drinkers of coffee were Sufis in fifteenth-century Yemen – coffee was felt to be a way of communing with God, and as it became a more widespread tradition over the centuries, ritual followed with it. One of the hardest parts of transitioning to this new pandemic life is the lack of coffee, such a vital part of so many of our day-to-day rituals, but new traditions have sprung up to take their place. Human beings are infinitely adaptable.

Saying my goodbyes to Julie, I get changed and head back upstairs. The ward feels unsettled – Kevin has normalized and Ali is improving. Maurice's niece has come and chatted to Dr Lam already, a rare face-to-face with a family member. Maurice is holding steady too – no better, but no worse. We spend the rest of the night fighting fires – smaller, but constant, emergencies to attend to. By the time morning comes, Maurice is still hanging in there. We hand him over to the day staff, relaying the grim picture he painted overnight. I stumble into a cab 40 minutes later, intent on working on a charity presentation, but drift off watching the central London streets slide by in the morning sun.

. . .

Remarkably, when I return to shift that evening, I'm delighted to find that Maurice is doing well. The day team, possibly due to a miscommunication, proned him anyway, and he has started to turn around. As a last-ditch effort, the day consultant started a high-dose steroid as well, which has been suggested to help in some of these long-term COVID patients. I hope Maurice improves, but it's a waiting game now. On our rounds he is on his front and will stay there until the morning. There is little to change.

Ali has not deteriorated further, and Kevin has also been started on steroids in the hope that he might be able to move forward. There are some new patients, including a desperately sick 81-year-old who appears to have suffered a heart attack during his COVID illness; he is rapidly fading despite maximum treatment, and the day team have designated him as "not for resuscitation", after discussing with his family the very low likelihood of their being able to restart his heart or lungs in the event that either were to stop working. Sadly, he passed away almost immediately after handover.

Another patient, a 41-year-old who has been transferred from another ward, deteriorates suddenly around midnight, and is moved back to the high-acuity intensive care to start on the direct blood oxygenation machine, ECMO. Despite those initial concerns about futility, so far many of the ECMO patients are still going, and there is a general consensus that it is worthwhile. The night shift passes oscillating between long lulls, sitting in sweltering PPE, and pant-wetting life-threatening emergencies, for which I still feel very unequipped. I'm just doing the best I can, as is everyone around me, and we're all simply hoping it's enough.

· · ·

The day breaks and we hand over, and I trudge out into the sunlight. Like coming out of a sauna, the air is cool and refreshing, and I feel meditative as I wander toward the car. Yet the world is silent, and as I walk past deserted underground stations and empty markets, I feel a sense of *jamais vu*, observing sights that I've known for years but no longer seem to recognize.

I'm not very good at emotions. It feels like things happen, sometimes difficult and stressful things, and I internalize them, but I'm blind to where those moments go. Sometimes I couldn't tell you how I am actually feeling, as if the inner and outer spheres don't connect well. I tend to not be angry or stressed when expected, and then every few months or so can unexpectedly boil over, sometimes over very little.

As I pull the car out of the car park, morning light filtering through the fresh spring leaves, I feel light and positive. But I wonder if this is simply the veneer, the lie that I keep telling myself to just keep getting through it, piling more and more in to avoid confronting the frustration, the fear, the stress and the long days and long nights in the dark tunnel of COVID ICU. When I was at medical school, I read *House of God* by Samuel

Shem, the semi-autobiographical traumatic experience of a first-year medic starting in a large US hospital in the seventies. When the protagonist rotates into intensive care, he experiences an epiphany, seemingly coming out of his depressive stupor and enjoying his work. But it is a façade – he hasn't dealt with his internal sphere at all; he has just created a new shell around it, uncoupling the work of looking after humans from his own humanity. I wonder if I'm doing the same, as perhaps we all are: getting through it, throwing myself in as much as possible, but with somewhere deep down all of that well of emotion building, biding its time.

CHAPTER 8

Recovery

The night before our wedding day, in my parents' garden, I wrote my groom's speech at 2 a.m. on a trestle table after a gruelling 16 hours setting up a venue for a hundred people from scratch. This might seem last minute, but at the pace we planned the wedding, this was par for the course. Finding it nearly impossible to get an agreed two weeks' mutual leave while rotating as junior doctors, we finally managed to find some time together with just eight weeks' notice. We decided to just plump for a simple registration, with very few guests, and then spend our meagre savings on a honeymoon. Needless to say, this plan did not go down well with either side of the family, so we found ourselves trying to plan an entire wedding in just under two months. "If you ever want to feel truly loved," my speech opened, "try to organize a wedding in eight weeks." I'm reminded of this feeling nearly every day as we try to set up and run a charity in the midst of a pandemic. By the end of April, we are edging closer to £1m raised. There's a feeling of camaraderie, of absolute unity of purpose with nearly everyone we work with. Every conversation is pushing on an open door and all the blood, sweat and more than a few tears are finally producing some returns.

．． ．

I'm sitting at my patio table on a sunny Wednesday morning, in what has become colloquially known as "my office". The powder-blue wrought-iron table has become my desk, the heavy trellis feeling reassuringly cool against my elbows. The table had been a labour of love – it took me months to get round to cleaning, fixing and repainting it, mixing two shades of metal paint to make a baby blue colour that Dilsan had asked for. I'm terrible at DIY, so any job takes me weeks of thinking about, and hours of consumed concentration, but a lasting and deep satisfaction with the result. A reminder that it was all worth it, in the end.

I'm working my way through my share of the charity calls, trying to catch up on the piles of clinic paperwork outstanding, when an email lands in my inbox. It simply reads "Innovative, sustainable and reusable PPE". We get perhaps a dozen of these emails a week now, mostly from companies looking to sell to the charity. This one catches my eye, as it's from a plastic surgery registrar called Yash Verma, from Oxford. It's a long email and I can't quite get what exactly the project is, but there's a video link at the bottom and I click through. The video starts playing, and it's suddenly crystal clear what the project is: a modified full-face snorkel mask attached by a 3D-printed conduit to an anaesthetic filter, the same filters we have been using at work to filter bugs and bacteria out of the ventilation systems. Our current FFP3 masks can last up to four hours before they need to be disposed of, and up to 70 per cent don't fit anyway. This mask is the opposite – a snorkel mask already designed to be comfortable and air-tight, attached to a filter designed to last up to a month at the low pressures of a regular person breathing. The potential is truly life-changing – a single GP or surgeon could wear this mask, changing the filter once a month, and never get infected. In some developing countries, a hundred of these masks might protect every medic in an entire region.

I think of all the colleagues that have lost their lives in the pandemic already, colleagues like Kevin lying in our intensive care units right now, so many GPs, nurses and surgeons, the impact this might have. If it works (it's a big *if* and subject to extensive testing), we could protect everyone, indefinitely. I feel nearly embarrassed calling Yash immediately after watching the video.

"This is revolutionary. This could change the whole crisis, especially for healthcare workers."

Yash just laughs. "Yes, we are rather fond of it too, and thanks for getting in touch."

"How did a group of plastic surgeons come into making respirator masks for COVID?" I ask.

Yash tells me the whole wild story. Based at the John Radcliffe Hospital in Oxford, their group are all plastic surgeons, the entire department, in essence. Growing frustrated with trying to operate in the current PPE, they started toying with the idea of making their own mask, an idea that spilled out into designers, developers, engineers and a fundraiser for £100,000, of which they've only raised £27,000 to date.

"Plastics making plastic," I say, laughing.

"You couldn't make it up," Yash replies.

I pause.

"I feel like I owe you an apology," I say.

"How so?"

"I saw this before, but it just didn't register. If I'd known about it, we wouldn't have spent so much time…" I trail off, thinking of the time we've already lost. "Anyway, let's get it safety tested and then on people's faces as soon as possible."

"Okay, so in terms of money…"

"We'll fund it. We can divert some of our legacy fund; it's better to stop colleagues dying in the first place."

"Quite."

We agree to get their product into the testing house ASAP, and then cross all our fingers and toes. This is a project that could change the world. A glimmer of hope in the dark tunnel.

· · ·

That weekend (24–26 April), I'm back on call, in one of the new intensive care units. It's oddly better set up than the original one – the bays are wider and the open windows pour in golden views of the London skyscape in the afternoon sun. The doctors' areas are not quite as well adapted, we hand over in a tiny repurposed office, 10 of us in a space designed for three. Dr Jansen is the consultant for the weekend. We've not worked together before but he's bright, cheery and thoughtful. As we start going through the handover, it becomes apparent that something has changed: the diagnoses remain the same – COVID pneumonia – and the number of days each patient has been here is significantly longer, 40 days on average, but the majority of patients are actually awake. Most have breathing tubes in their neck now, and a couple are planned for further insertions in the week. We can communicate with them and a few are even close to discharge from intensive care.

Ali is one of those – after spending weeks on the ventilator, his numbers on our little paper handover sheet are finally starting to turn, and he's even managing an hour or two a day breathing on his own. "COVID, it turns out, is a marathon," Dr Jansen intones, as we remark on several of the patients finally improving, after months in the unit. It might be a good day after all. But it seems we spoke too soon, as the crash call goes off for bed 8. My heart sinks as I realize it's Ali, slumped in his bed, the saturation probe now flashing close to 70 per cent, which is dangerously low. We boost the flow of oxygen coming through the ventilator and try suctioning the tube, pulling up bloody clots of mucous. Dr Jansen passes me the stethoscope. I listen to Ali's chest; one side gives a whisper in and out with each breath, while the other makes no sound at all. I examine his chest, wrapping each hand around the side of his ribs and leaving the thumbs free in the midline – this is how we assess the amount of air going into each lung. One hand moves, but the other doesn't. This indicates that one of Ali's lungs is blocked, the main airway plugged with mucous or a blood clot, and he is struggling to manage on one already-damaged lung alone.

After more suctioning and repositioning, Ali seems to be recovering again, but he is up and down like this all morning. We've seen this before, a sign that Ali's failing lungs may not last much longer. Dr Jansen disappears from the ward to conference with some of the other consultants. He comes back full of determination.

"Okay, let's 'bronch' him," he says.

"Bronch", or bronchoscopy, is a procedure where a long tube with a camera on the end is inserted into the windpipe and then into the lungs themselves. Using this, we can see a blockage and even suction it out. The problem is that it's also one of the highest-risk procedures in generating aerosols, the most infectious particles. We have been generally avoiding doing bronchoscopy on any of the COVID patients for this exact reason. Also, I'm still not sure it's going to help Ali.

We clear the room as much as we can, and only essential staff for the procedure stay in. The tube snakes down the tracheostomy port and immediately locates the problem, a large blood clot in the main airway to the left lung, the left main bronchus. Dr Jansen manages to tease it out, but Ali isn't tolerating the procedure at all well. His saturations drift down, and before we can do anything else, his pulse wave on the monitor dissolves into a flat line.

"Cardiac arrest," Dr Jansen says, calm and collected. "CPR."

The charge nurse starts CPR, and we slap the emergency pads on him from the crash trolley as it comes wheeling in.

"P.E.A.,"* Dr Jansen calls. "Adrenaline."

I crack the box open and pass the glass vial of adrenaline to the nurse at the line, who fiddles with the IV and pushes the whole drip in, in one go. We continue CPR for two minutes and when we stop, we see a rhythm again. Ali's breathing is better again as well, and there's definitely air going into that lung when we re-examine.

---

* Pulseless Electrical Activity

"Keep him flat today – we will see how he goes tomorrow."

We're all hoping he finds his way through this latest episode – he's been through so many highs and lows. We update his family, but their responses are quiet – they've heard all this a dozen times before. We finish the ward round and I realize that every patient has been here for more than four weeks. It also strikes me that we don't have any new patients – perhaps things are plateauing. There isn't much to do after the ward round, and we spend the afternoon checking in on Ali intermittently and tidying up admin jobs.

Wondering if this is the peak of the crisis, I message Hugo and ask how the Nightingale is going. His message is blunt in reply.

"Haven't done a clinical shift yet! Wonder if I'll be back before I ever do!"

It sounds like the Nightingale Hospital is in a similar position – the pandemic seems to be levelling out and cases mercifully starting to fall again. There's a long lag time, however, and plenty of work still to do.

We hand over the patients that evening and go home. On my walk back to the car, the streets are still deserted. I think of Ali, his months on the ventilator, and all of the others, some far more unwell. I wonder if we will see an end to the marathon soon. It feels like a glimmer of hope is starting to appear.

* * *

The next day starts well, and gets better and better. Thankfully, Ali is nearly back to normal the next day, a little drowsy, but his ventilator settings are back to where he was the day before and he is alert enough to even talk a little. He gestures to his chest and mouths the word "sore". Understandable, given the chest compressions just the day before. We increase his pain relief, and he rests.

The next patient is Jacob, a 60-year-old retired civil engineer. He's been in the ICU for 35 days and has very much been through the ringer. He's been ventilated for weeks, proned and deproned, suffered infection after infection, kidney failure, liver failure, undergone a tracheostomy, began bleeding and suffered another infection. But slowly he started breathing for himself, spending longer and longer off the ventilator, until, a few days ago, he didn't need the ventilator at all. The tracheostomy came out, and now here he is, very weak but able to talk and even eat a little. He's ready to go to the ward. He's the first COVID patient I've physically discharged from intensive care and it gives me pause. I feel something inside me lightening. We check him over very carefully, going through his charts and medications and bloods, examining his lungs and heart. He's been through an incredible amount, but here he is. Bright and alert, and even chatty, as far as he is able, his voice still very strained and feeble, having had a tube between his vocal cords for nearly a month. When I tell him that he can be discharged today, he just goes stony silent. I'm not sure he understood me. I repeat it but he just nods, not saying anything at all. I think he needs some time to process all this. I think we all do.

And then, a few hours later, I call the ward to give a handover about Jacob, who has just arrived there. By coincidence, the registrar who picks up the phone has just seen him.

"How is he?" I ask.

"He's quite emotional really, very grateful. He keeps saying 'I shouldn't have survived'."

That hits me hard, somewhere deep. I take a breath.

"I guess they all just need time in the end."

Suddenly feeling the need for a cup of tea, my hands on fire again, I ring off and organize a quick break with the team. Peeling off the PPE, I wander into our rest area, slouch in a corner and quietly sip. It's an odd time for a break and the area is deserted, except for one of the coordinating nurses I've not met before at the front desk. She's humming to herself as she's drawing on something I can't quite see. I watch as she gets up, holding a paper star, and takes it to a board I've not noticed before in the corner of the room. There are many, many other stars there. She pins up hers, and I can clearly see it says "JACOB" in big wide letters.

I recognize some of the other names on the board from previous shifts, none of whom I knew had been discharged. I had assumed they hadn't made it. At the start of the pandemic all our data suggested that so many of our patients, more than half, would not survive, that there was little hope. And yet, months later, here was the proof, a whole constellation of hope incarnate. The board is a testament to the dedication and skill of my colleagues, a testament to the institution. I'm sure there are similar boards all over London, and the country. We've turned a corner. The world feels a little lighter again.

• • •

I bump into Nat again later that same day – we haven't seen each other in months, splitting onto different rotas very early on and rarely crossing paths. She's been doing the follow-up clinic, calling up the discharged patients at home and seeing how they are. Of the five she called today, I've looked after two, Khalid and John. They are at home, with their families, still weak, nowhere near 100 per cent, but they are there. They still have their small complaints, aches and pains that Nat can do little but reassure them about on the phone. Give it time, she tells them.

The first ever major heart attack I saw was a middle-aged man, who came streaming into our heart attack centre a few minutes from death. Halfway through the procedure to open the blocked artery in his heart, with long catheters threaded through his wrist, carefully manipulated inside the heart vessel itself, his heart trace suddenly disappeared in a storm of erratic electric impulses, a fatal heart rhythm called ventricular fibrillation. We shocked him on the table twice and then carried on. The boss fixed his artery, and he woke up half an hour later, and was fully recovered and eating chicken korma on the ward that evening when I went to see him. The only thing he had to tell me, a man who was technically dead a few hours before, was that his tooth hurt. I advised him to see a dentist at some point. Sometimes it's the small complaints that might be the surest signs that patients are on their way back to their normal lives.

· · ·

We move another patient into Jacob's bed, christening it the "lucky" bed, which may be more than a superstition, as it faces a wide-open window and the tips of a tall oak tree wave back and forth in the sunlight. As a motivating, uplifting view I can't imagine much better. We hope the next patient will do as well as his predecessor. By the end of the weekend Ali is fully recovered. I was far more sceptical about his chances, but Dr Jansen just keeps repeating the same thing: "It's a marathon, not a sprint." Maybe the finish line is coming into view.

· · ·

Two weeks later, I'm on my way upstairs to another shift when I bump into Hugo in the foyer of our hospital. He's back from the Nightingale. His hair is shaggier, somehow underlining the fact that it's been months since we last saw each other. It's a nice reunion, although there is no hand-shaking or hugs. I wonder if there ever will be again.

"So, what was it like?" I ask him.

"I missed it," he says.

"What do you mean?"

"I was on the rota, but never got called in. There were only 50 patients there in the end."

"That's good, isn't it?"

"It is, I guess." Hugo shrugs.

"It's good to have you back, anyway." We both smile at that as I head upstairs, on my way to another shift.

A little early, I wander around to that same board of discharged patients. There's a new little star, in the front and centre of the board. It simply reads "Ali". He just needed time, and that's exactly what everyone here has worked tirelessly for – to give him the time his body needed.

I look for other names: Maurice, Jeffrey, many more. Missing. To some extent we will carry some patients around with us for years after we meet them. It's part of the doctor–patient process, a process that leaves a footprint in the head and sometimes in the heart. Their faces and stories, conversations with loved ones, all of the connections that add up to how we as doctors construct our patients' lives, how we remember them.

· · ·

A month later, we're into June, but the sky is a cold-grey steel with a threat of rain. Ayla is dashing back and forth to the living-room shutters. We are waiting for some very special guests, the first guests to come near the house for months. A car pulls up on the road outside, and Ayla squeals with delight.

"Teyze, teyze, Adam! Emir!" she shouts, running headlong to the door. Dilsan and I are waiting at the doorstep, waiting for Nesli. We've set this up ahead of time – chairs over two metres from the house at the top of the drive, and chairs for Dilsan and Ayla on our doorstep. We've synchronized the snacks so the kids can all eat the same things. Nesli is carrying a bag of goodies for her boys, Adam (three) and Emir (five), as they clamber out of her car. Dilsan and I are both just about holding it together, but being reunited with Nesli and the boys after weeks and weeks is overwhelming.

The boys look so grown-up and don't try to run toward us. Having shielded for months, they are well trained in the dangers of the "germs". Ayla has had the same spiel but is still trying to run to her cousins, and even Zach is trying to crawl across the drive.

"Nesli!" Dilsan calls to her, her voice thick with emotion.

"Hello, guys. Missed you." Nesli is flushed, similarly over-whelmed. Her boys are a little shy at first and shuffle onto the chairs. That shyness soon disappears, though, as we move on to our planned social distance party activities: a dance-off. The boys are on their feet, and Ayla is shouting to her cousins to check out her moves, all respecting the two-metre divide. Zach is trying his hardest to crawl onto the dance floor. What a strange time for these kids to grow up in, I reflect. They soon tire, and we tuck into the snacks. Ayla keeps calling to them to make sure they are eating the same crisps or fruit that she is – it's a sweet way of sharing an experience from further away than usual. Emir is asking when we can play chess – I taught him just a few weeks before the lockdown and he picked it up crazily quickly, but we haven't had a chance to play again.

"Soon, Emir," I call back.

"When the germs are over, Emir!" Ayla calls to him.

Emir is happy with that. He gets on with his snacks.

"When will that be, though?" Nesli asks.

It's a strange time – cases are flattening out, yet the number of cases and deaths are still far higher than anywhere else in Europe, and we have started unwinding the lockdown already. At work for the past fortnight we hadn't had any new transfers and have slowly begun the laborious process to wind down the intensive care units again and get back to normal life. And yet, with Ehsan at home still shielding, and with it being advisable to continue to shield as much as possible for the foreseeable future, I wonder about the risk of mixing properly like we used to. We have more cases right now than we did when we locked down.

"I'm not sure anyone knows, really, Nesli," Dilsan suggests.

"I guess this is the new normal," Nesli replies. "For now, at least."

We put the music back on for the kids, watching their distanced dance-off. Adam is dancing furiously, lost in his own world, and all of them are laughing and shouting.

"It's not so bad," I laugh.

For now, at least.

Epilogue

IMMUNITY

This book was written in and of its time, in a sea of ever-changing facts, science and new data. Every time we look back at what has become the greatest crisis in a generation, there will be more to learn, more to see. Sitting here right now, looking back at the UK's response, all I can see is devastation.

As I'm frequently reminded, I am neither an epidemiologist, nor a virologist. I have no expertise in any of these fields other than what has rubbed off on me over the years. I am a doctor, armed with Google and a napkin. I would claim expertise in one field, however, and that's NHS capacity, resource and funding – it's an area I have spent years of my life studying, campaigning in, and writing about. On Dilsan's and my honeymoon, I wrote a 5,000-word treatise on the junior doctor contract; at a friend's wedding, I created and edited a viral visual essay on the NHS, with a heavily pregnant Dilsan in the background giving me pointers; and I staged a rally to support the NHS on one of my own birthdays, as it was the only day we could book an outdoor space large enough.

At every stage in my relatively short career in medicine, it has been obvious on the ground that the effects of a decade of cuts, pay freezes and closures could be truly catastrophic. As one of my registrars used to put it in my first year working as a doctor, "as one A&E closes, another one is f**ked". When I've tried to draw attention to this simple fact, of the self-harm inflicted by consistently supporting measures that result in a depleted workforce with diminishing morale and resources, it has been like shouting into an abyss, shouting myself hoarse. Pictures of a sick child lying on an A&E floor during the run-up to the December 2019 general election weren't enough to sway hearts and minds, so I'm not sure why I ever thought my voice would make a difference. The simple numbers are so bad they speak for themselves; at present, we have the worst A&E waiting times on record, the worst operating wait times and the worst record on hitting cancer targets. Even life expectancy is on the decline. We are short-staffed by a figure of around 100,000 staff, including 40,000 nurses. We also have one of the lowest number of critical care beds, general hospital beds and doctors per head of all the 37 countries in the Organisation for Economic Co-operation and Development (OECD). If we were an army, we would be a band of bedraggled, starved and exhausted soldiers. And that was all the case before any sign of coronavirus.

The only thing we ever knew about COVID-19 for certain was that we didn't know much about it; it is a brand new virus, from a very mixed family of viruses, ranging from common cold-like viruses to deadly respiratory syndromes that have already killed thousands in recent epidemics. What was immediately obvious was the body count – a visible, tangible number of dead. We can argue about case fatality ratios and infection fatality ratios for years, and likely will, but what is unarguable is that people, in their hundreds and thousands, were dying. And this was not only readily apparent from the initial outbreak in Wuhan, but also from the *Diamond Princess* cruise ship, and from Iran, Tenerife and Italy. We could see the pandemic unfold, in high definition, live, 24/7, before our very eyes. And yet, for too long, we did nothing at all.

Although I don't believe in "isolation fatigue", the idea that people will simply get bored of imposed lockdown measures, I can understand it in principle. I think it's a tragic underestimation of the fortitude and resilience of the British public, but I can understand the thinking behind it, however flawed. What I can't understand is why the government took no unilateral measures to curb the spread: providing hand gel and hand-washing stations at transit hubs, disinfecting trains, quarantining flights from at-risk areas and banning mass recreational gatherings. These were all measures that were imposed in other countries. The medical community was already cancelling its conferences anyway, and it speaks volumes that we decided to do this independent of any government advice. A colleague of mine flew from Lombardy on the very day they went into national quarantine, and strolled through Heathrow airport with nothing to declare, going to work the next day as a busy London GP. No one seemed to think this was a problem. God only knows how many similar stories there are.

On the ground, waiting for coronavirus to appear in our London hospitals, I saw first-hand the complete lack of preparedness. Physically, we didn't detect the early community cases at all, and couldn't test the ones we did, inadvertently letting the virus infect patients and staff with impunity. We didn't have sufficient PPE, and our winter preparedness stocks were out-of-date and were insufficient anyway, without any plan to mobilize them in a timely manner, should the need arise.

Mentally, we weren't prepared either – that threshold into the pandemic world was hard to see and harder to cross. The only thing worse than suddenly having to deal with a once-in-a-lifetime crisis is not being told about it, not being able to take the time to mentally prepare. We will be facing the prospect of a generation of healthcare workers traumatized by that alone.

The titanic effort from the NHS to suddenly rally round, cross-train staff, expand units, sweep away all the bureaucracy and admin that had kept us from being so effective for so long and just get on with it was a privilege to behold. A colleague of mine had complained for three years about a clock that was screwed onto the wrong wall in her anaesthetic room, so it couldn't be seen while intubating a patient, when the seconds are vitally important to keep track of. The same hospital built a 16-bed resuscitation area in their A&E waiting room in three days. It was always possible. But why were we so pressed for time, when that tidal wave of disaster was so vehemently visible, when we could *see* the bodies in the streets in Wuhan, the patients in the corridors in Lombardy, the endless warnings, from the WHO, from *The Lancet*, from public health experts and behavioural scientists and thousands of others? I remember telling Hugh Pym – the BBC News Health Editor – to think of this as the Blitz, and he looked at me like I was a crank. And yet here we are, well past the Blitz death toll of approximately 43,000 now.

The lockdown came late, and, as some SAGE* scientists are now coming forward to say publicly, this came at the cost of thousands and thousands of lives. How many GPs, surgeons, nurses and even transport workers were thrown under that bus, inadvertently exposed while the government assured us there was no community spread, and then stopped testing entirely when there was, against all pandemic guidelines anywhere? What would Ehsan and Nesli have been doing if they didn't have medical relatives to advise them to do something differently to the government advice? The paternalistic, opaque, callousness of the government approach is infuriating and demeaning.

Was this always the plan? Was the government planning to try and produce "herd immunity"? The pieces of the herd immunity narrative are strewn through the last six months and paint an ugly picture. On 3 February, Boris Johnson gave a speech at Greenwich, claiming one country should "make the case for the right of freedom of exchange" and prevent unnecessary measures that were "beyond medically rational". He described "some country ready to take off its Clark Kent spectacles and leap into the phone booth and emerge with its cloak flowing as the supercharged champion … I can tell you in all humility that the UK is ready for that role."† Later, in conversations with the Italian Prime Minister, Boris Johnson was on record as stating "herd immunity" as his goal.‡ The position of his chief

---

* The UK's Scientific Advisory Group for Emergencies

† https://www.gov.uk/government/speeches/pm-speech-in-greenwich-3-february-2020

‡ https://www.independent.co.uk/news/uk/politics/coronavirus-uk-boris-johnson-herd-immunity-dispatches-channel-4-italy-prime-minister-a9544916.html

special advisor, Dominic Cummings, was reportedly summarized at a private function in identical terms: "herd immunity, protect the economy, and if some old-age pensioners die, so be it" – although the fact that he said this was subsequently denied. Chief Scientific Adviser Sir Patrick Vallance described "herd immunity" as useful as late as 13 March,* despite his own admission that it would require 60 per cent of the population – around 40 million people – to become infected. With the 1 per cent fatality rate proposed at the time, that would equate to around 400,000 dead. A death toll like we have never seen in this country, but one that seemed to be the goal.

Perhaps the gamble was that the virus would turn out to be far less deadly than thought previously, with many more asymptomatic patients, and therefore far fewer deaths were it to pass *en masse* through the population. A gamble indeed, one which many other countries would not partake in: New Zealand and South Korea locked down very early and suppressed the virus. A gamble, at least to date, that history will look unkindly on, as we approach 70,000 excess deaths, the number of deaths above the five-year average for this period. That's an Old Trafford-size football stadium full of men, women and children, gone. Was herd immunity ever a valid game plan? To allow the virus to take hold, to reach the high levels of deaths we have seen, in order to protect the economy?

Well, firstly, there was no evidence, and remains no evidence to date, that being naturally infected with COVID-19 even definitively confers immunity to subsequent infection. We aren't

* https://www.youtube.com/watch?v=2XRc389TvG8

sure it happens at all. I took my antibody test, a government-backed reliable version, and it was negative. We've had colleagues who tested positive with the swab test but went on to have negative antibody tests. We have family who were all living together and all were sick, but one has positive antibodies and the other two don't. The reliability of these tests is in doubt, but a gamble that infection would mean lifelong protection was a colossally unsure one.

Secondly, herd immunity by natural infection has never happened in the history of mankind – it's only been achieved by using a vaccine. But with this crisis, vaccines were discredited as taking too long to be a viable solution. A vaccine is the only realistic way out of coronavirus, and never has there been a more pressing need to produce one. The entire world is focused on that problem, to apply the whole gamut of resource and skill of a globe of human beings, and that would inevitably lead to much quicker delivery of a vaccine, or other treatments, than in normal circumstances. To date, the only treatment that has evidence to back up its effectiveness against coronavirus appears to be a steroid, called dexamethasone, a class of drugs we have been using for decades in intensive care, and indeed were already using in many of our patients long before these study results were announced. Further trials will come, and much sooner than for any previous condition. We won't have long to wait on that, and I pray that by the time you read this a vaccine is widely available.

Thirdly, if you infect 40 million people you will quite quickly realize that the age spectrum of severe disease is wide, and stretches right down to people in their thirties and even younger. I looked after patients as young as me in our intensive care. And no, they didn't have significant "underlying health problems". Reports of a post-viral inflammatory syndrome in children, and fatalities in babies and children, suggest that the initial sense of relief that children were untouched was short-sighted. Worse, we are yet to see the long-term effects of post-viral infection, a whole litany of symptoms of chronic breathlessness, weakness and fatigue. Had we infected millions, or if we still intended to, what long-term effect might that have on the workforce? We would be the sick man of Europe anew.

Lastly, there was the argument that delaying the lockdown was supposed to protect the economy. The government's rationale here was predicated on the belief that closing down shops and pausing or ending livelihoods may eventually cost lives in the same way, through economic deprivation, crime and poverty.

Workforce damage to the younger population aside, the best analogy to explain why this was a spectacularly stupid idea is to imagine the virus as a fire. Exactly like a fire, it grows and multiplies in the right conditions at an exponential rate, and, left unattended, it will burn your house down. When you find a fire, the longer you leave it, the larger and hotter the fire burns, and the harder it is to put out. Similarly, throwing a blanket over the fire early will smother it, but closing a door on a blaze will only dampen it, and the fire will be ready to explode back to life when that door opens again. Countries that locked down early took a small economic hit, perhaps as little as a week or two more of reduced activity, but then had far fewer cases to deal with, could wrangle that case burden down quicker, and came out of lockdown with far fewer residual cases to have to trace, contact and continue to suppress. In contrast, we allowed our epidemic to peak far higher and, confusingly, decided to start to come out of lockdown with the rest of the world, when our cases and our deaths were still that much higher than any in Europe. We are much more likely to struggle to control our case numbers and therefore end up with a second wave far sooner, experiencing lockdown and its consequent economic damage all over again, not to mention another colossal, if not worse, death toll, as a result. Our own estimates in the OECD suggest that not only have we suffered the worst death toll, we will also suffer the worst economic insult as well. The worst of both worlds.

The tension between "economic" and "viral" deaths is, however, a false one. People losing their lives in a society where there is no safety net of support, education and financial security is not an inevitability – it is a failure of government imagination and a choice of fiscal policy. Just like the policy of austerity in 2010, which chose to cut public services, was not an inevitable consequence of global recession, and some would argue was in fact the opposite of traditional economic theory. Death from a global pandemic of a deadly virus is immutable – there is little anyone can do to avoid this once you are infected. So to mitigate loss of life, the choice is between the very difficult and the impossible, and that's no choice at all.

We have talked constantly about not "overwhelming" the NHS, and even some pundits now look back and say we weren't "overwhelmed". Let's be very clear: we absolutely were. We had to triple or quadruple the number of intensive care beds and had to divert all staff away from their regular jobs. We cancelled nearly all of our regular activity, much of which involved looking after very sick people and making them better, because we had to look after a whole new deluge of incredibly sick people. That first group didn't go anywhere – if anything, many would have got worse – and will now languish on spiralling waiting lists. And we did nothing to protect the most vulnerable in our care homes, letting them die in their thousands, even reportedly discharging patients with COVID-19 directly to the sector. We now know that COVID-19 in the elderly can sometimes be very mild and unusual, presenting with confusion, falls, abdominal symptoms or sometimes nothing at all. We didn't bring those patients into our hospitals and that's where they died. We didn't have capacity to cope with a mass pandemic – hospitals had to close wards and even entire A&Es due to a shortage of beds and oxygen supplies. Hundreds of healthcare workers died. The narrative that we simply "coped" is a dangerous and insulting fiction, an insult to the monumental effort and sacrifice the service had to give to save as many lives as possible.

Every step of the way the government has been guilty of a total lack of transparency. From the earliest rationale of why we diverged so far from the WHO and the rest of the world's mantra of *test, isolate, track and trace*, as well as shunning other measures like lockdown far later, it was never clear what the modelling was to guide these decisions. To take such a drastically different direction without obvious reasoning could only invite disaster – disaster that could have been avoided with public scrutiny. Worse, the government narrative of false reassurance led to the double-effect of increased spread, as the public didn't take the threat seriously, and incredible trauma, as hundreds of thousands of people lost loved ones without any adequate warning, without any chance to prepare, to protect them. Despite pleading that the government followed "the science", this was never shared with us. And later on, we learned that political aides had attended scientific meetings – to what end if not to influence them?

When the lockdown came, I hoped that would be the end of the failings, but it was only the beginning. That lethal combination of incompetence and mendacity shone through in fiasco after fiasco. Take PPE, for example. The government denied there was a problem, then downgraded the requirements rather than attempt to increase the supply and protect staff properly, failed to find a logistical solution to get stocks to where they were needed, and then let large-scale purchases go by the wayside until it was too late, suddenly finding themselves making deals with Turkey to buy token amounts of PPE, and then lied about there ever being a record of that purchase. Even worse, they awarded PPE budgets to companies with no capability or experience of producing PPE at all. A single patient requires 30 sets of PPE *per day* in an ICU. France ordered *2 billion* masks for their healthcare workers in April, while official government stats showed that the UK had only ordered a quarter of that number by the end of June.*

Testing was a similar fiasco, and in particular stopping community testing entirely on the grounds of it being "pointless". It was the only way to control the epidemic at a time

---

* https://www.newstoday.fr/france-has-ordered-almost-2-billion-masks-from-china/?utm_source=rss&utm_medium=rss&utm_campaign=france-has-ordered-almost-2-billion-masks-from-china; https://www.bbc.co.uk/news/health-52254745

of exponential rise, but the government refused to change the guidelines for hospital patients for days when it was evident that community transmission was well established, leaving unknown cases to infect staff and others. It then became obvious that we lacked the large-scale capacity to keep up with the pandemic, setting dodgy targets and dubiously meeting them through double-counting, before finally deciding to stop reporting the number of actual people tested entirely. The government spent £12 million on an app for contact tracing, but then, when it didn't appear, we were told it would never have worked, and, again, diverged from the global standard. On a government level, we couldn't have managed any aspect of this crisis worse, and appear to have learnt absolutely nothing from it, jettisoning our scientific advisors and disseminating confusing messaging to the public at the critical moment when coming out of lockdown could explode in our faces. Throughout all of this, the government displayed a basic lack of humility, failing to acknowledge and correct these mistakes as they were discovered, and an insane focus on public relations as opposed to public health policy.

On the ground, it's a very different story. Whatever we thought going into the pandemic, the truth of it has been lived, experienced and absorbed. There's no denying or running away from it. I've never been prouder to work in the NHS than during the last few months. I saw the very, very best of my colleagues, contorting to a Herculean degree to bear the weight of this crisis on their shoulders. Colleagues suddenly thrust into positions of life-or-death responsibility, workloads doubled or tripled to organize rotas, expand services, write guidelines, build new A&E departments, even source millions of masks for their own unit from China. Nurses parachuting into the no-man's land of intensive care, terrified in unfamiliar territory, and yet there they were, sleeves rolled up, ready to help.

So what have we learnt?

One, with the right mindset, we are capable of incredible things. We swept away bureaucracy and administrative chaff and were led by pure clinical need – hospitals moved internally like a Rubik's Cube at high speed, building units, throwing up resuscitation areas and going above and beyond, and just kept going and going. It'll be that much harder for good ideas to be shouted down as impossible when we've all witnessed this.

Two, we know a lot more about coronavirus now than we did going in. It's a nasty, sticky, strange disease and, close-up, looks more like an autoimmune process at the severe end, with multiple systems including kidney, lung and heart involved. Steroids might help in very sick patients, and while many other treatments don't appear to work very well at all, repeated proning seems to be effective. Fundamentally, what so many of the severest patients need is time – it's a marathon of weeks and weeks of ventilator time, and escalating to the highest level of therapy is justified to get them that time. How we build that into our capacity-planning for the future, keeping extra intensive care beds and staff ready and waiting, will be key to managing the next wave.

Three, we need to value and support our staff. Around 50,000 NHS staff will leave the service each year, under normal circumstances. Retention was a major issue *before* any of this started, and a recent survey conducted by the Institute for Public

Policy Research estimated that up to 300,000 staff plan to leave the service at the end of the pandemic. Even if only a third of that number actually follows through, we are looking at a catastrophic future loss of the most vital healthcare resource we have: people. In a country with comparatively very few healthcare professionals per head, it's a precious resource we cannot afford to squander. The measures to support the wellbeing of staff cannot be withdrawn now, they are needed *more* in this time after the first wave if we want to build a workforce capable of getting us through the next one. Not to mention the huge backlog of work we have waiting for us, with up to 10 million people expected to be on waiting lists by the winter of 2020. Sorting out the healthcare service could take a decade or more, and the work will only get harder. Morale and retention measures are cost-saving in the long run, not an unnecessary frivolity, and we must recalibrate to that. A widespread culture change, to build in mental health support and counselling, is equally important; there will be large swathes of staff left demoralized, depressed and even traumatized. We need to keep every single one.

Lastly, having learnt new ways of doing things, it seems impossible to return to the old ones. Telephone clinics, for one; calling patients at their home, at their convenience, is better for all parties, it would seem, at least in the short term. Similarly, how we use our healthcare resources, resources that were already stretched and now will be far further stretched trying to catch up, will need to be carefully rationed. Sending patients to specialists without due cause, specialists following up with patients for no reason for years, unnecessary imaging tests, this will all need to end. We have all got much closer to having walked in each other's shoes now, and hopefully those experiences will make us a better team, less siloed, more cooperative.

Unpicking this litany of failures will be an inquiry of its own and will take a decade or more. When the human body is invaded by a pathogen, a complex cascade of cellular responses isolates, neutralizes and breaks apart the foreign material, "presenting" the debris to specialized cells that can then produce the immunoglobulin, or antibodies, that will make the response faster next time. The body breaks down a threat into its constituent parts, antigens, and studies each one, to better prepare and defend itself in the future. We need to do the same urgently. Whether it's the second wave of COVID-19, a new coronavirus, or another pandemic in the near future, this *will* happen again unless we learn the lessons that we are being presented with right now.

Everything we did before the pandemic seemed alarmist, inflammatory. Voices calling to heed the WHO guidance, calling for an earlier lockdown, people like Richard Horton, editor of *The Lancet*, and Lord Ashcroft, former director of Public Health England, were sidelined as dissenters and sensationalists. That must've been difficult to take – I know because I got more than a few of those accusations myself, for speaking out in public. Even at the time, and shortly after the fact, I wondered if it was the right thing to do, if there was a better or less inflammatory methodology. But then, what would you have done? If you had genuinely convinced yourself that the national conversation would lead to an unprecedented loss of life, a colossal death toll unheard of outside wartime, and even then eclipsing the Blitz, what would you do?

The "duty of care" that doctors have, to speak up on behalf of their patients, is a complex one. On the one hand, we must prioritize patient safety at all times, and "must take prompt action if you think patient safety, dignity or comfort is being compromised".* On the other hand, whistleblowers and patient safety advocates have found themselves ostracized or even the subject of a modern-day "witch-hunt" when raising concerns.† There's a tremendous amount of politics and focus on reputation that clouds the ability to listen when things are going wrong. This needs to change, from the top down. I, and many others, came to the conclusion that trying to do so something in the face of such a potential catastrophe was better than doing nothing.

When the human body is pushed beyond its natural reserve to oxygenate and supply blood to exercising muscles and tissue it switches to a different, less efficient, form of energy production to keep going. This is anaerobic respiration, "without air", and the by-product is the build-up of lactic acid in the blood, which can cause dizziness, breathlessness, muscle ache and fatigue. It takes the liver some time to effectively metabolize the build-up and return the body back to a state where it can be fighting fit again.

As a college student I signed up to the Duke of Edinburgh Gold Award. I'd never gone orienteering in my life, didn't do much exercise, was generally very lazy, and thought I would just pop along for a 50-mile trek over two days with no problem at

---

* https://www.gmc-uk.org/ethical-guidance/ethical-guidance-for-doctors/raising-and-acting-on-concerns
† https://www.telegraph.co.uk/news/2020/01/17/hospital-demanded-fingerprints-doctors-hunt-whistleblower-inquest

all. By the end of the first day, having trekked 20 miles across the soggy south Wales hills, my legs, back and arms burned. I remember sitting down heavily on my pack at the campsite, just staring at the ground, my legs simply gone. I couldn't move them. It started to rain, thick, heavy, summer drops: the life-giving weather of the Welsh valleys. My team, already peeved with me for struggling to keep up, were now staring in disbelief as I just sat there, getting soaked to the bone, simply unable to move, trying to metabolize that lactate build-up. Eventually they got me into the tent, and I slept through from that afternoon to the next morning.

All of us, inside and outside the NHS, have been running on full steam for months, well beyond our normal reserves. In the health service, we were already running on fumes, with the longest waiting times on record, and now we have had to push past that to cope with the pandemic, but all of those waiting lists and backlogs, that lactic acid, is still here.

The pandemic has been a fundamental challenge to so many of our societal norms. Home-working for one, decreased use of air travel and travel in general for another. While pollution of the air and the waters may have decreased in turn, we need to be more attuned to the dangers of information pollution, the streams of misinformation, conspiracy theories and organized bot networks that promote actively harmful behaviours. The facts are deadly important in a pandemic, and we have already had mask-deniers, 5G towers being burnt and death-toll hoaxers. If we are to grow as a mature society, we need to clean up the endless white noise of online and offline charlatans and quackery. We need to demand that same integrity, that same credulity from those in power – so far, we have consistently chosen the opposite, and that has led us to disaster. We must learn from the pandemic – all of this cannot be for naught.

The pandemic isn't over. The first wave has passed, the waters are receding. The virus hasn't gone away, and as we come out of lockdown with such a high case number, we shouldn't expect it to simply disappear by itself. It will only be by the actions of the public, everyday people like yourself, that we can hope to control it, to prevent a second or even a third wave. The basic advice will always be the same: avoid unnecessary gatherings, wash your hands, work from home if you can. Whatever the rhetoric, you have lived that experience now of what the pandemic was like at the coalface, and understand more than most what is at stake.

. . .

I've had the same recurring dream since childhood. I'm standing on a beach, looking out, staring at the blurry haze where the pearl-blue of the sky and the deep green of the sea merge. Along the beach are dozens of families: fathers, mothers, sisters, brothers, cousins, grandparents, partners, sons and daughters, all doing the same.

Standing together, watching the horizon.

Addendum

After the events of this book, a singular life event happened that I suppose it would be remiss of me not to discuss.

In May 2020, newspapers reported that Dominic Cummings, chief special advisor to Boris Johnson, had broken the lockdown rules at the peak of the first wave. As it later emerged, Cummings broke the guidelines on three separate occasions: not self-isolating when his wife became ill and returning to the heart of government probably infectious himself; driving 250 miles at an uncertain time point, when he was symptomatic, to self-isolate on his elderly parents' farm; and finally, driving 30 miles on his wife's birthday to a local beauty spot at Barnard Castle, to "test his eyesight", going in and out of various areas before driving to London. "Barny castle", incidentally, is local Durham slang for a "pathetic excuse".*

There has been no single intervention in human history that has saved more lives than the lockdown. Uncontrolled viral

---

* In the sixteenth century, the expression "That's Barney Castle!" became associated with a cowardly excuse after Sir George Bowes, who was steward of the castle, barricaded himself inside it, refusing to come out to fight during the Northern Rebellion of 1569 (a failed attempt by Catholic nobles to oust Queen Elizabeth)

spread was predicted to kill over half a million people in the UK. The lockdown measures were a social contract – we all agreed to limit our own personal freedom to protect ourselves and our loved ones, and by extension everyone else's loved ones as well. It was a social contract that inflicted huge personal cost on the entire nation: closing businesses, separating loved ones, cancelling weddings and letting many die without their loved ones at their side. Yet it was that social contract that controlled the pandemic, saved hundreds of thousands of lives and protected as many staff in the NHS as possible from being completely overrun and infected themselves.

The issue here was not the transgressions of a single wayward special advisor – it was the subsequent farcical circus of nearly the entire Cabinet and the Prime Minister lining up to defend him, to pretend there was no breach of the lockdown, even to rewrite the rules in retrospect, to tear up that social contract as if it wasn't important. The only thing that can get us through this pandemic is trust and transparency, and in a single weekend the government burnt both to a crisp.

On a Sunday afternoon at the end of May, coming back from a break on ICU, I tweeted an angry photo of myself in full PPE, stating that if Dominic Cummings didn't resign, I would. Why did I do this? I suppose it's a question I will likely be asked for the rest of my career, so here is the bluntest and most honest answer: I was bone-tired – in body, in spirit, in soul. For months, we had been trying to do anything and everything to contribute to the relief of the pandemic, at work, at home, through the charity and SHIELD. As a family, as a workforce, as a country, we were giving everything to get through the pandemic. This wasn't an imposition, this was the deal, the fundamental contract: we all give up a little, or sometimes a lot, in the name of something bigger, to protect everyone. And it was working. I had seen first-hand for months the consequences of the virus, and the eventual difference the lockdown made. The beneficial effect of the lockdown was tangible to us in the NHS, perhaps in a way it wasn't tangible to many others.

It wasn't the nonsensical movements of a special advisor that incensed me – it was the government response, the attack on the credibility of the lockdown, that contract that had saved so many lives, that so many had sacrificed so much to uphold. All for the sake of an apology, which is all it would've taken. Some token acknowledgement of wrongdoing, to acknowledge and maintain the importance of the lockdown. Instead we got Cabinet ministers and then the Prime Minister pretending there was no breach, despite the facts to the contrary, and a subsequent fairy tale about a castle and an eye test. They even laughed about it.

This was not okay. This was not just another government indiscretion we could shake our heads at and accept. Prioritizing public relations over the risk to hundreds of thousands of lives was unacceptable. In that fatigued moment, after everything, it felt like a punch to the gut. Vindictive and cold. Personal to me, to so many of my colleagues that felt the same. If the ultimate decision-makers in the country could be so flippant, so insultingly callous in dismissing our efforts, for the sake of nothing, then what was the point of all of this?

There has to be a line of what we will and won't accept. This cannot all have been for naught.

To be honest, I never dreamed that Cummings wouldn't resign. My optimism and faith in the world is a real blind spot and so often misplaced these days. If he'd simply apologized, I would have accepted that, had the good grace to back down. All I ever wanted was for the lockdown to be respected and its credibility preserved, the social contract protecting all of us upheld. I never thought I would watch an hour-long trashing of that contract in the rose garden of Number 10 Downing Street.

When it became clear that this was where the government had pitched their tent, lying to the face of the entire country, rewriting the rules of the lockdown in spirit and letter to contort around one single person's inability to simply apologize, I initiated the process to resign. I believe very strongly that you should say what you do, and do what you say. That straightforwardness is missing from every part of our national conversation and I can't stand it. My supervisor was very disappointed. I got more than a few messages of support, even one or two job offers, and one or two colleagues who took a dimmer view. After talking it over with Dilsan, I resigned my training number and position, working the remainder of my notice for three months in intensive care, figuring that if a second wave came, I would be needed here.

After the tumultuous period settled, I felt free. I love being a doctor, it's part of my make-up and my being and will always be who I am. There are also plenty of parts I don't love, however: the faceless, administrative, tick-box nature of modern medical training, the politics, the bravado, the bullshit. I felt incredibly sad to leave cardiology behind, but, frankly, there are other ways and means, perhaps more impactful ways, to make a difference. Perhaps we will cross paths again some day.

I have spent years trying to effect change, to make the country a better place for my kids and family, but also for everyone out there, campaigning for the NHS, trying to educate the public, trying to correct the poisonous narratives that dominate our national conversations. But that's all it ever was, conversation, just words. Crying to myself helped no one, did nothing.

And then we did something different, moved from negative criticism to positive action, and reached out into the world to effect positive change with the charity. I hope my sparking off on television led to some small changes somewhere, words that fell into receptive ears and changed a few minds, perhaps, but those aren't visible to me, or tangible. What is visible is the hospice that stayed open, the junior doctor emotionally grateful after her first counselling session, the medical student with a place to stay and finish her studies, and all of the rest. We did all we could. Even in failure, that brings a peace of mind and soul that Twitter threads never did.

Looking ahead, the first wave was exactly that, only the first challenge we faced. The challenges to come – a second or even third wave, a global recession, climate change, mass misinformation and disinformation, and political and societal upheaval on a generational scale – will all require more from all of us if we hope to meet them. The challenge of our generation is not behind us, it is only just beginning. I plan to continue doing something about it, and perhaps now you do as well.

So stay informed, stay safe and be kind.

Acknowledgements

So many thank yous:

To Dilsan, for everything, for always.

To Beck, for never letting me give up, and for giving so much.

To Mum and Dad for supporting me 100 per cent, always.

To Nej, also known as Obi-Wan, for making our ramblings reality.

To the 'Brogues for never letting my head get too big.

To the whole HEROES team, past and present: Michelle, Jack C, Ed, Kyri, Kate, Ellie, Ravi, Ray, Will, Justine, Jess, Jeeves, Jon, Jack T, Sem, Caroline, Chloe, Nikki, Kim, Issie, Antonia, Nic, Simon, Steve, Mike, Nick, Imogen, Jem, Maddie, Kate O and Sade.

To SHIELD and Paul, Nigel, Tim, Nate, Jacob, Maxine, Phil and James for your brilliance, commitment and eternal drive to help.

To Max, without whom there would be no author.

To Oli and Nathan, without whom there would be no book.

To all my colleagues in the NHS and the wider healthcare sector, thank you for all that you do and continue to do.

And to all the patients I have had the privilege of knowing and caring for. You taught me as much about medicine as about life itself.